Walk It Off

Walk It Off

Make Pounds Disappear the Easy, No-Fail Way

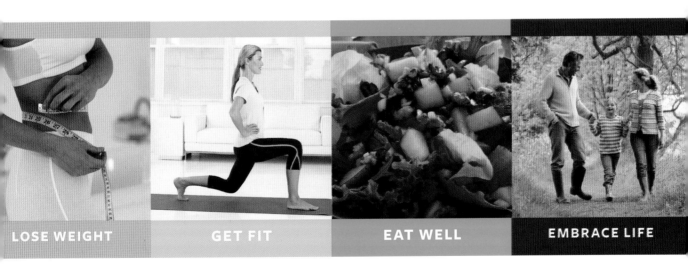

LOSE WEIGHT   GET FIT   EAT WELL   EMBRACE LIFE

Reader's Digest

The Reader's Digest Association, Inc.
New York, NY/Montreal

Project Staff

Consulting Editor: Karen Watts

Editor: Barbara Booth

Designer: Rich Kershner

Cover Designer: Jennifer Tokarski

Reader's Digest Trade Publishing

Senior Art Director: George McKeon

Executive Editor, Trade Publishing: Dolores York

Associate Publisher, Trade Publishing: Rosanne McManus

President and Publisher, Trade Publishing: Harold Clarke

Library of Congress Cataloging-in-Publication Data

Walk it off : Make pounds disappear the easy, no-fail way. -- 1st ed.

p. cm.

ISBN 978-1-60652-359-9

1. Walking. 2. Weight loss.

GV199.5.W355 2012

613.7'12--dc23

2011028445

We are committed to both the quality of our products and the service we provide to our customers.
We value your comments, so please feel free to contact us.

The Reader's Digest Association, Inc.

Adult Trade Publishing

44 South Broadway

White Plains, NY 10601

For more Reader's Digest products and information, visit our website:

www.rd.com (in the United States)

www.readersdigest.ca (in Canada)

A NOTE TO OUR READERS

We pledge that the information and advice inside *Walk It Off* has been checked carefully for accuracy
and is supported by leading health experts and up-to-date research. However, each person's health, fitness,
and healing regimens are unique. Even the best information should not be substituted for, or used to alter,
medical therapy without your doctor's advice.

Printed in China

1 3 5 7 9 10 8 6 4 2

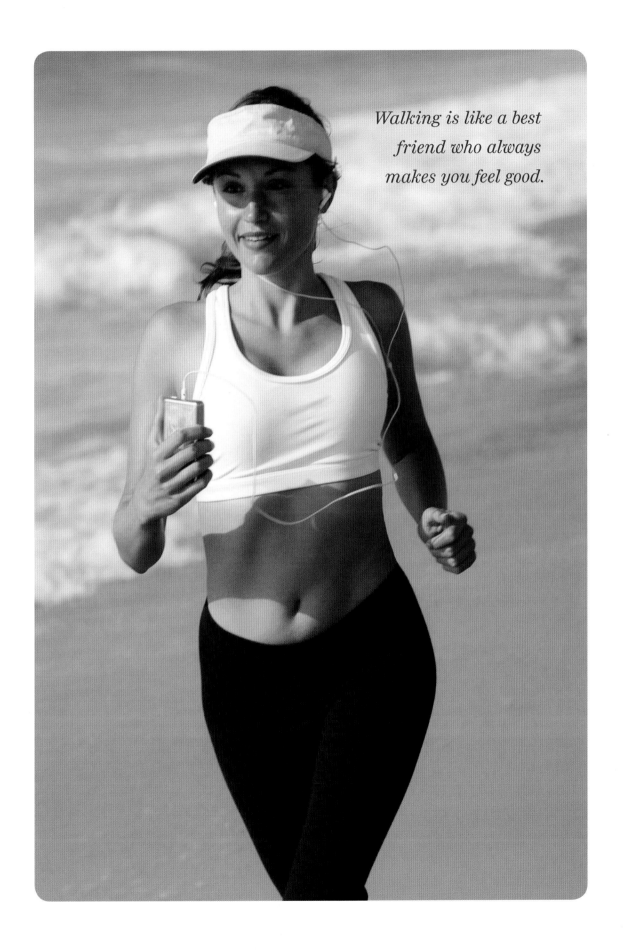

Walking is like a best friend who always makes you feel good.

Contents

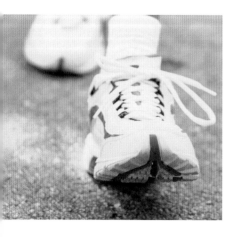

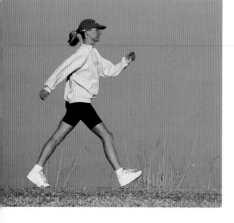

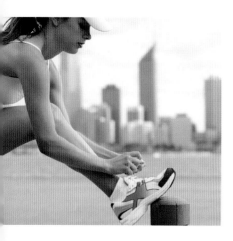

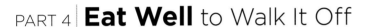

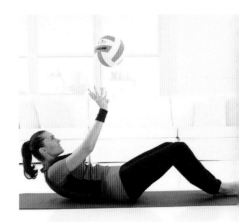

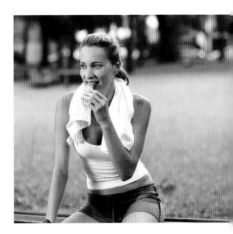

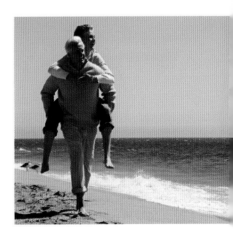

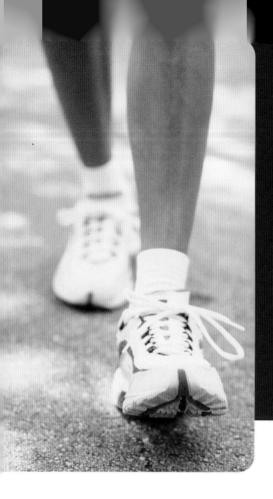

Introduction

Intuitively, we know being fit is a good thing.

It feels great, gives you energy, and makes life's tasks so much easier. But is exercise really crucial to weight loss? Isn't it really just about how you eat? And if exercise is so important, what type and how often?

You'd think that the scientific community would have come to some agreement on the answers to these questions by now. But they haven't. Many widely held "truths" about fitness have been proved wrong in recent years, replaced by fascinating new insights many doctors aren't even aware of. The good news: Recent studies show that the right type of fitness for health and weight loss is much more within our reach than we realize.

The fact is, fitness is a critical part of the weight-loss equation, and there's only one practical, effective way to achieve and maintain a healthy weight: Move more and eat less. Or move more and eat better, to be precise. And by move more, we don't mean become a triathlete or train for a marathon. We just mean *move more*.

That's because your body is meant to move in natural, ongoing ways, as our ancestors did. Breakthrough research from recent years reveals that active daily living—frequent short walks, taking the stairs rather than the elevator, regular stretches and movements, routinely picking up and carrying things—is healthier for you than short, intense workouts surrounded by lots of sitting. Who would have thought that the ticket to fitness and good health would be the ordinary day-to-day stuff—you know, *life*—that doesn't require loads of time, fancy athletic wear, or an expensive gym membership? Go figure.

That's where walking steps in. Simply putting one foot in front of the other repeatedly throughout the day is the world's most perfect form of exercise. You can do it anywhere, anytime, and it requires nothing but your own two feet. It's convenient, social, inexpensive, low impact, and most important, fun! And besides being a proven fat-burning, metabolism-boosting, weight-loss tool, active walking also reduces stress, clears your head, increases energy, improves your sleep, and just generally brightens your outlook.

With all these great benefits, how can you lose? *Walk It Off* provides the inspiration you need to jump-start your routine, along with hundreds of tips and tricks to make your workout more effective and keep you motivated. In this book you'll find:

- The skinny on why walking works
- Ready-to-go walking programs for new walkers, seasoned walkers, and everyone in between
- Strength-training exercises designed to build muscle and burn fat
- Stretches to warm up, cool down, and improve flexibility as you get stronger and more fit
- The inside scoop on the power foods that will give you energy, stabilize your blood sugar, and help you succeed in your weight-loss goals
- A month of Walk It Off menus, featuring delicious power food–rich recipes
- Practical, new advice on how to outsmart bad eating habits
- Out-of-the-box ways to think about walking any time of day, every season of the year
- The best places to walk from sea to shining sea
- Cool walking gear and gadgets that'll kick your routine up a notch
- And much more

This book will stretch your limits, flex your muscles, and streamline your diet so you can quickly lose the weight and achieve the body you were meant to have.

Ready to get started? Come on. Let's take that first step together.

THERE'S ONLY ONE PRACTICAL, EFFECTIVE WAY TO ACHIEVE AND MAINTAIN A HEALTHY WEIGHT: MOVE MORE AND EAT LESS.

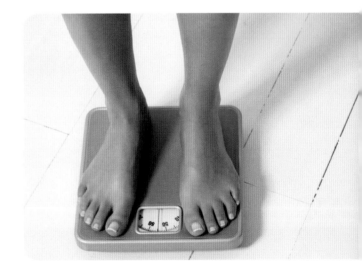

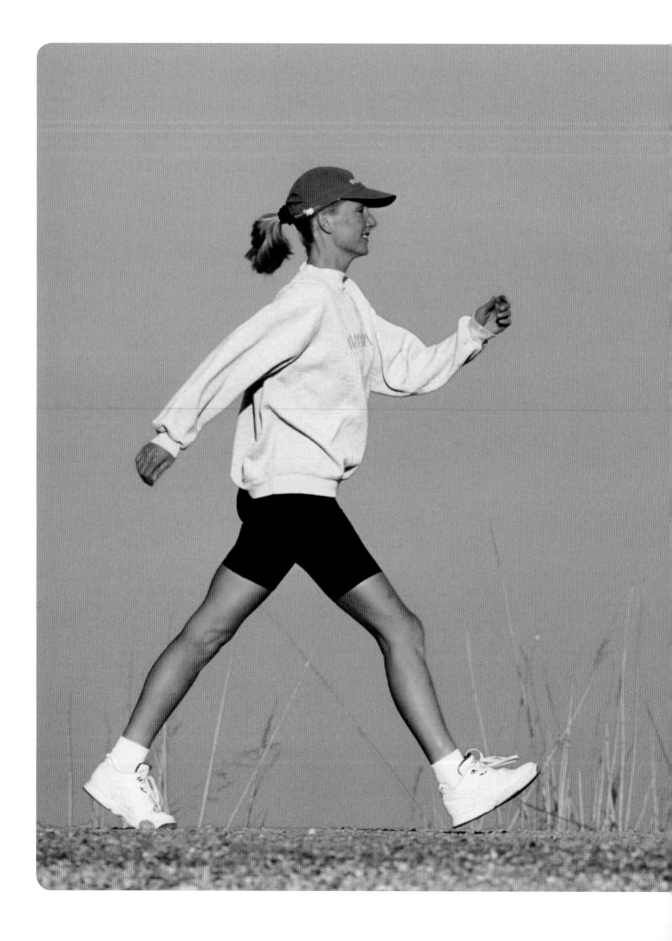

Get Ready
to Walk It Off

WALKING REALLY IS AS SIMPLE AS putting one foot in front of the other. So if that's all you do, you're already way ahead of the guy on the couch eating chips and watching *The Godfather* weekend marathon! But if you really want to get serious about walking off those extra pounds, you need to think differently about walking. Not only is it important to appreciate the dramatic physiological transformation that happens to your body when you walk but also to realize the consequences that can ensue if you don't walk. And in order to get maximum weight-loss benefits, you also need to understand what exactly your body should be doing when you walk. How you walk, how long or how fast you walk, where you walk, even when you walk can make a difference in reaching your fitness goals.

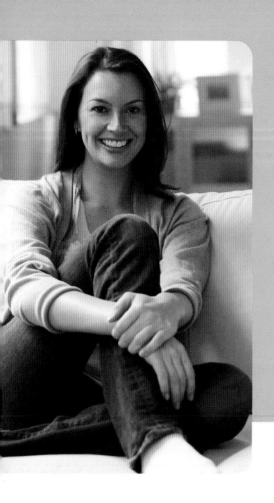

Why Walking *Works*

Imagine a "miracle vitamin" guaranteed to help you drop a clothing size or more; banish blue moods; serve up more shut-eye; slash your risk for heart disease, diabetes, and cancer; and spice up life in the bedroom. Did we mention that it's also perfectly safe and costs virtually nothing?

You won't find this super supplement in any pharmacy, but you can easily pick it up on the way to the store. It's vitamin "W"—walking. The perfect dose? Hit the sidewalk (or the trail, treadmill, or mall) for 30 minutes most days of the week. There's no need to own a killer outfit, spring for an overpriced health club membership, or waste time (and gas) driving to the gym.

But is exercise really crucial to weight loss? Isn't it really just about how you eat? And if exercise is so important, what kind and how often?

You'd think the scientific community would have solid, agreed-upon answers to these questions. But it doesn't. Many widely held "truths" about fitness have been proved wrong in recent years, replaced by fascinating new insights many doctors aren't even aware of. The good news? Recent studies show that the right type of fitness for health and weight loss is much more within our reach than we were led to believe.

A Brief History of Weight

Scientists believe humans have been on this planet in its current form for roughly 1 million years. For 999,940 of those years, no one but athletes and warriors bothered to exercise. They didn't need to. Most of their waking hours were spent carrying, tilling, building, or battling with enemies. This kept them fit. Another plus? No fast-food restaurants or boxed cookies. Food was scarce, given the lack of refrigeration and electricity. Needless to say, this kept them lean.

This epoch ended only about 60 years ago. In the past six decades, thanks mostly to technology and industry, food not only became plentiful but food businesses discovered that the more sugar and fat they put into their products, the more people enjoyed them. Some of that is animal instinct; our bodies are naturally drawn to high-calorie foods as part of the self-preservation process.

At the same time, we became sedentary. Television, computers, desk jobs, Internet shopping and socializing, long commutes by train, bus, or car.... It seems that life has conspired to keep our bottoms attached to our seats. Here again, animal instinct is at play: Our bodies are naturally drawn to rest as part of the energy-conservation process.

Put it all together—much less movement, much more food—and you have the underpinnings of the modern obesity epidemic.

Now, some scientists will talk about an "obesity gene" that makes certain people (in the United States nearly half of the population with European ancestry, according to one account) gain weight. Forget it. Even if you were to have a "fat gene," it's not your DNA that makes you pack on weight. It's how you live today.

HERE'S THE SKINNY ...
Our current obesity epidemic is easily explained by dramatic shifts over the past few decades toward abundant calorie-rich food and a lifestyle dominated by sitting.

Staying Slim in Today's Times

So how do we maintain a healthy weight in these modern, high-tech times? There is only one effective way: Move more and eat less. Not one or the other, but both. Adjusting only one rarely works. Merely eating fewer calories won't compensate for all the sitting we do. And no level of exercise can burn off all the empty calories in the typical diet. The remedy? A gentle, slow adjustment to both your eating and movement patterns.

You probably know the basic rules of eating for weight loss. But how do we adjust our lives to get in adequate fitness? Usually, the wrong way. For several decades now the government, scientists, and a huge fitness industry have been telling us to put on workout clothes and get physical. At least three 30-minute sessions per week, doing some precise mix of weight lifting and aerobic exercise. There's no surprise, then, that roughly 80 percent of Americans choose not to exercise.

And even when we try it, it doesn't work. Let's paint a picture. Someone—let's say you—resolves to lose weight once and for all. You know you need to exercise, so you

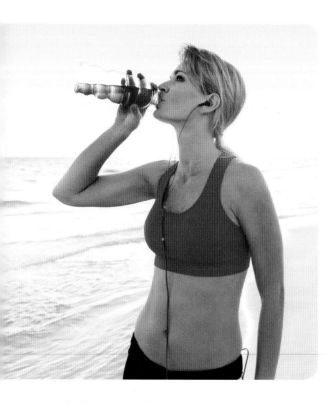

start jogging. You've heard you have to be properly fueled and hydrated, so you drink a Gatorade and hit the streets. But jogging is hard and leaves you feeling sore and punished. Regardless, you go for it, and afterward you feel you deserve a reward. So you stop by Starbucks and treat yourself to a pumpkin scone. Four weeks later (if you make it that long) you haven't shed an ounce and despondently toss your running shoes aside.

What happened?

First, you treated exercise as a special, additional activity rather than a natural part of your day. Second, you chose an activity that is too challenging, particularly for someone who hasn't been exercising. The result? Your workout was short and painful and left you feeling totally spent. Yet you burned only the caloric equivalent of an ounce or two of weight. The Gatorade and snack more than compensates for the calorie burn, effectively washing out your workout.

Your body is meant to move, so you should move it. But in natural, ongoing ways, as our ancestors did. Breakthrough research from recent years reveals that active daily living—frequent short walks, taking the stairs rather than the elevator, regular stretches and movements, routinely picking up and carrying things—is healthier for you than a short, intense gym workout counterbalanced with lots of sitting.

The new fitness paradigm is to move a lot in ways that are fun and natural. No clothing changes or drives to the gym, just active daily living. Don't make it a chore. Just get out of your chair and move, as often as you can.

The next level of fitness? Movement activities that you'll enjoy, like walking, swimming, biking, hiking, golf, or tennis. Things you did for fun with friends when you were younger. Do these on a regular basis and you'll return to the physically active lifestyle of our lean ancestors.

And unless you're doing these activities on a competitive level, you don't need energy drinks, power bars, or any other special food before, during, or after. Just be active and eat normally, and weight loss with follow.

HERE'S THE SKINNY...
Active everyday movement restores the optimum daily balance between calories consumed and calories burned.

5 Health Dangers
You Can Walk Away From

You may have heard already that walking lowers high blood pressure, improves cholesterol ratios, and bolsters bone health—already more value than any single prescription medicine or treatment can deliver. Now a growing stack of research is adding important new benefits to the list. Simply putting one foot in front of the other can help you overcome these five big hidden health threats.

Sitting disease

In one study of 37,000 people, researchers discovered that sedentary living—going from bed to car to chair to couch, as so many of us do—is now a bigger killer than cigarette smoking. Walking is the natural cure for sitting disease, slashing your risk for lethal threats like heart disease, stroke, diabetes, and cancer. Just a half-hour jaunt every day cuts heart attack risk by 30 to 40 percent, report Harvard Medical School researchers.

Visceral fat

The fat you can't see is the most dangerous kind. Packed deep inside your belly, around your internal organs, visceral fat is now known to drive diabetes, heart disease, high blood pressure, stroke, and a host of other health conditions. Dieting alone won't make it budge, but walking will. In a recent Wake Forest University Baptist Medical Center study, women who walked 1 to 2 miles three times a week shrank abdominal fat cells by a whopping 18 percent in four months. Conversely, these dangerous cells remained packed with fat for women who dieted but didn't walk.

WALKING LOWERS HIGH BLOOD PRESSURE, IMPROVES CHOLESTEROL RATIOS, AND BOLSTERS BONE HEALTH.

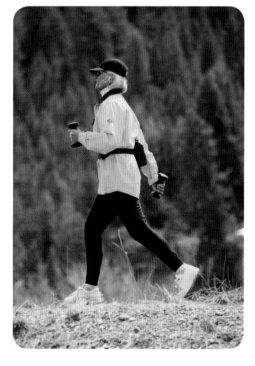

Extra pounds

Slashing calories may help you squeeze into that size 10 dress for your high school reunion, but research proves what anyone with a closetful of "fat" and "skinny" clothes knows: Dieting won't help you keep pounds off. What does? You guessed it. In one ongoing study of 4,000 people who've successfully maintained a 30-pound weight loss for a year or more, 78 percent walk. (Hate diets? Strolling for 20 minutes a day could help you lose 14 pounds in a year, report scientists from the University of Missouri–Columbia. That's a better return than most weight-loss programs!)

Insulin resistance

Added pounds and inactivity conspire to make tens of millions of us develop this silent condition in which the body grows deaf to insulin, the hormone that tells cells to absorb blood sugar. Insulin resistance raises your risk for diabetes, heart disease, Alzheimer's, and a host of cancers, but the best treatment isn't a drug. In one landmark study of people with insulin resistance, walking reduced the odds for developing type 2 diabetes by a whopping 58 percent. (A diabetes drug cut the risk by just 31 percent.) Walking lowers blood sugar immediately, because muscle cells drink it up. It also makes cells more insulin-sensitive for hours afterward.

Stress

Chronic uncontrolled tension keeps levels of cortisol and other stress hormones sky high for days, weeks, even years. The result: more headaches, sleepless nights, digestive upsets, depression, and high blood sugar. Research shows that walking combats 24/7 anxiety by boosting levels of feel-good brain chemicals like serotonin and dopamine, by easing muscle tension, and by giving you a mental break from your worries. It's no wonder that in one recent eight-year-long Temple University study of 380 women, regular walkers said they felt significantly less stressed than non-exercisers. In another study walking helped sleep-challenged people nod off 15 minutes sooner and gain an hour of shuteye per night.

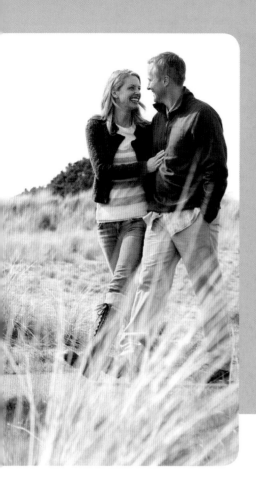

How to *Maximize* Your Walk

Walking acts as an appetite suppressant and helps build muscle. It feels great, gives you energy, and makes handling life's tasks so much easier. But to optimize your fat-burning strategy, you need to prime your mind, your heart, and your muscles and understand that when you eat is as important is what you eat.

Get Your Head in the Game

In the handful of minutes it takes to watch the evening news each night, you could be whittling your waist—as well as slashing your risk of diabetes, stroke, and hip fracture. You could also be improving your mood, sharpening your thinking skills, and getting a better night's sleep. The only thing holding you back from reaping these big-time benefits is . . . well, you.

Your attitude about walking is the key to being the trim, fit, healthy person you want to be. If you put it off until you feel like exercising, forget it. Waiting for the perfect wave of enthusiasm to lift you off the couch and out the door just doesn't work.

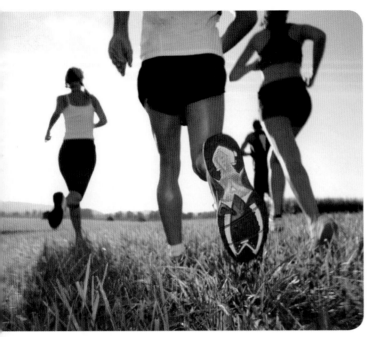

Instead, clearly identify your objective and commit to a schedule to make it happen. Write down your weight-loss goal and post it on your fridge and on the bathroom mirror so you're reminded constantly of your aim. And schedule time in your calendar every day to walk. Once you get walking, you'll see that rather than being something you dread, walking will become the pound-reducing, head-clearing, rose-smelling highlight of every day.

Increase Your Aerobic Activity

So now you've learned that ongoing movement is better for your health and weight than short, intense workouts alone. But that doesn't mean you should rule out exercise. For weight loss, building in some intense movement to your week makes total sense. What's changed is what that exercise should be.

Aerobic (that is, fat-burning) exercise literally means "with oxygen." Any exercise that raises your heart rate and gets you breathing a little harder (but not gasping) recruits what are known as your slow-twitch muscle fibers. These fibers make the energy you need by taking stored fats (as well as some carbohydrates) and blasting them with oxygen in the mitochondria, your cells' furnaces.

When you push beyond your comfort zone, those slow-twitch fibers fade like over-loaded fuses, and your body calls in the backup generators—your fast-twitch fibers. These fibers go straight for your glycogen—or stored carbs—and blast away without oxygen (anaerobic). The result is an instant power boost. Lifting weights is an anaerobic exercise because it calls for short, intense periods of exertion. This method of energy production creates metabolic waste, which causes your muscles to burn and fatigue.

The more fit you are, the faster and longer you can walk, swim, or bicycle before going into the "red," that zone described above in which your muscles start to cry uncle. The point between aerobic and anaerobic is called your lactate threshold. To condition your body to stay aerobic and burn more fat—which is what you want in order to lose weight fastest—you need to raise your lactate threshold.

Doing that is a simple two-step process. Part one is spending the majority (about 80 percent) of your exercise time in your aerobic zone. Your body will respond by cre-ating more capillaries to deliver blood to your working muscles, as well as beefing up your mitochondria, so you'll be able to push yourself a little harder and longer while still burning fat and staying aerobic. Second, you want to condition your body to work harder so it "resets" that lactate threshold point, making you burn more calories from

BRIEF PERIODS OF MORE INTENSE EXERTION CAN TURN A LEISURELY STROLL INTO A WORKOUT.

fat in a wider range of exercise intensity. The best way to do that is to exercise using intervals. During a walk, swim, bike ride, or other aerobic activity, simply pick up the pace (or turn up the resistance or incline on your stationary bike or treadmill) until you're breathing and working pretty hard for about 30 seconds. Then go easy for a minute to 90 seconds. Repeat this cycle five or six times. Twice a week of intervals is all it takes to greatly increase your fat burning!

HERE'S THE SKINNY...
The best exercise for weight loss is an aerobic activity like walking, biking, or swimming, with several short bursts of full-out exertion mixed in.

Make More Muscle

So now you know that to lose weight, you need to eat less and move more. Merely cutting back on calories won't compensate for our increasingly sedentary lives.

You also know that the most important activity is everyday movement. Walk more, move more, sit less. Lots of natural movement is the key to a healthy weight. And you know that once you are ready to add formal exercise to your routines, it's best to focus on interval training. It's the optimal way to burn fat.

So what's left? The next step up the fitness pyramid is strength training. Now, many people misunderstand the goal of lifting weights. To them pumping iron is either about physical power or body sculpting. And how many of us really worry about either of those? There's a much more compelling reason for us to have healthy, strong muscles than appearance. Muscle tissue burns three times as many calories as fat, even when you're doing nothing more strenuous than watching television. Muscles burn calories around the clock—yes, even when you sleep—at a greater rate than other body tissue. That's why you need to keep making and maintaining muscle as you age: to keep your body's ongoing fat-burning metabolic engine revved.

In fact, it's never too late to fan those flames with resistance training. One recent 12-week study found that men and women age 60 and older lost an average of four pounds simply by lifting weights three days a week, without changing diet or exercise— more evidence that lifting weights helps you beat the battle of the bulge, not make you "bulky," as novice weight lifters fear. Strength training also helps improve your balance and posture by strengthening the core stomach and back muscles. A small daily dose of focused muscle strengthening is all you need to stay toned, stand tall, and keep your calorie-burning engine in high gear.

HERE'S THE SKINNY...
Strength training builds muscle that increases metabolism to help you burn more calories around the clock.

Match Food to Fitness

Aerobic exercise most efficiently burns off the fat inside your body, which is the primary objective of weight loss. And as it turns out, by eating healthy fats, you train your body to be better at fat burning, too.

In a Harvard study of 101 men and women, researchers put half the group on a low-fat diet and half on a diet that included about 20 percent of calories from healthy monounsaturated fatty acids, or MUFAs. Great sources include nuts, avocados, olives, and safflower oil. Eighteen months later the MUFA-eating group dropped 11 pounds, compared to their low-fat eating peers, who shed only 6 pounds despite similar calorie consumption.

The message: Train your body to burn more fat by including healthy MUFAs in more of your meals and reducing your consumption of carbs and sugars. For optimal weight loss, roughly half your daily calories should come from carbohydrates; the rest should come from lean proteins and healthy fats.

Finally, when you eat can be as important as what you eat. It's repeated more frequently than *Seinfeld* reruns, but it's a fact: Breakfast is the key that turns on your fat-burning metabolism for the day. Research shows that people who skip their morning meal are four and a half times more likely to be overweight than faithful breakfast eaters. So instead of omitting the most important meal of the day, you should aim to consume about 25 percent of your daily calories for breakfast.

HERE'S THE SKINNY ...
What and when you eat can make you a better fat burner. Aim for more healthy fats, and consume a quarter of your day's calories at breakfast.

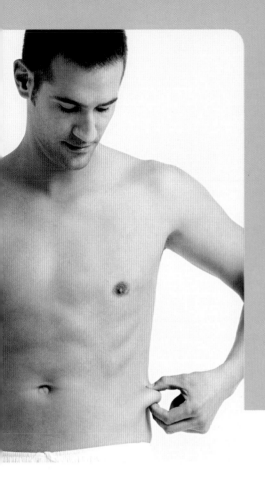

10,000 Steps to a *New You*

Gym teachers, athletic coaches, even the U.S. surgeon general have misled us. Over the years, they've conditioned us to think of exercise in terms of time and distance. How long was your workout? How many miles did you do? What's your best time for a 5K? Did you get the recommended 30 minutes of exercise today?

Think Small

What Americans need is a new, more inspiring way of quantifying activity. To keep from getting bigger, we need to start thinking smaller. Instead of measuring our exercise efforts in minutes and miles, we need to break it all the way down to individual steps.

This isn't a new concept. The American College of Sports Medicine (ACSM) and other fitness organizations have advocated taking at least 10,000 daily steps (about 5 miles) for years. Why 10,000? Studies have found that's the level at which you're burning enough calories to reduce the risk of obesity and chronic disease. But the concept hasn't been widely adopted, because most people either don't wear pedometers all the time or they don't have a clue as to what all those steps mean in everyday terms.

Here's a baseline to consider: People living completely sedentary lives take about 2,000 steps a day; non-exercisers on a typical day take closer to 4,000 steps. The ACSM classifies anything below 5,000 daily steps as sedentary.

Spend a couple of days wearing a pedometer and your perspective on exercise will change dramatically. It will make you more conscious of being active—walking down the hall to chat with a coworker rather than e-mailing her, doing errands on foot rather than in a car—and your concept of exercise will evolve from something you did for a specific time at a certain place (that is, morning at the gym, afternoon on the tennis court) to something we did all day, everywhere.

Experts now believe that a shift in focus from "working out" to "being active" is the key to getting fit—and staying trim—for life. In fact, researchers at the University of South Carolina estimate that women who are active 75 percent of the day (running errands, gardening, cooking, and so on) expend about 10 percent more energy overall than those who visit the gym for an hour but are sedentary the rest of the day (they sit at a computer). That's right—a day of housework can trump an hour on the elliptical trainer.

Spread It Around

Here's another way to look at it: Because we're so busy, most of us have put exercise in a box. Walking is something we do for a half hour before work or after lunch. It's separate from life—something that needs to be scheduled and worked around. Which means it will forever remain a chore or something easily bumped from our never-ending to-do list.

ALONG WITH COUNTING STEPS, SOME PEDOMETERS CALCULATE DISTANCE AND CALORIES BURNED.

To lose weight and keep it off for good, take exercise out of that box and spread it throughout your life. You can accomplish this by wiping the word "exercise" out of your vocabulary and replacing it with the word "activity." And you can do it by forgetting about minutes and miles and focusing on individual steps.

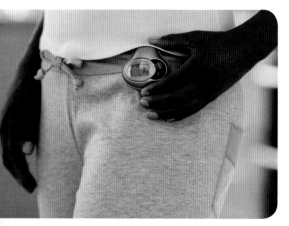

Buy a Pedometer

Here's what you're going to do: Head to your local sporting-goods store and buy a pedometer (less than $20). Put it on first thing in the morning and check it before and after doing . . . well, everything. Before long, you'll become a pretty good judge of how many steps you take doing your normal day-to-day activities.

Now start to think about how to increase the steps you take in an ordinary day. A rule of thumb is to increase your activity level only about 10 to 20 percent a week. If you're emerging from a winter of hibernation, consider yourself sedentary (taking about 3,000 daily steps) and add about 300 to 600 steps weekly. That'll not only keep you from straining yourself but also motivate you psychologically by conveying a sense of progress.

Note that it doesn't matter how long or short your strides are or whether your daily steps are taken uphill or down, indoors or out. For simplicity's sake a step is a step is a step. Note, too, that the following step counts are estimations based on anecdotal rather than scientific experience.

Target: 10,000

Here's how to begin looking at walking and exercise in an entirely new, potentially life-changing way. Add in a few of these activities and you'll soon discover that 10,000 isn't such a large number, after all.

First, figure out how many steps you're taking right now, without making any changes. Wear that pedometer around for a week. Put it on first thing in the morning and don't take it off until you go to bed. Note the number of steps you're taking each day in a log or notebook. At the end of the week, calculate your average daily steps. That's your baseline.

Once you have a good sense of how many steps you're taking (or not!) every day, begin to look for easy ways to beef up your step numbers by 10 to 20 percent. Think about your daily routine—morning chores, going to work, doing errands, family activities—and brainstorm the ways you can squeeze in more steps. Look for all the spots in your day when you could be walking instead of driving, walking instead of sitting or standing, and walking instead of using those contraptions—elevators, escalators, subways—that were invented so you wouldn't have to walk!

Continue to keep track of your daily steps in your log. Once you've succeeded in increasing your steps by 20 percent for a week, calculate the number of additional steps it would take to increase by another 20 percent. That's your next goal.

The 10,000-step strategy can get you looking at walking and exercise in an entirely new, potentially life-changing way. Add in a few of these activities and you'll soon discover that 10,000 steps isn't such a large number, after all.

- Park in the last row at work, the supermarket, or the mall.
- After parking, take the scenic route. Go around to the back door at work or use the farthest mall entrance.
- Never use the drive-through anywhere. Park and walk inside to do your business.
- Take the long way to the mailbox. Go out the back door instead of the front, and return the same way.
- Take the stairs throughout the day rather than the escalator or elevator.
- Take out the trash instead of hounding someone to do it.
- Walk around the house for 5 minutes making a honey-do list.
- Use the farthest bathroom from where you are sitting.

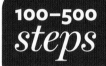

100–500
steps

- Walk the kids to a different bus stop. There's no rule that says you have to use the same one every morning.
- Pace while you talk on the phone, making it a rule to never sit down.
- Cook and serve dinner to your family.
- Chat face-to-face instead of e-mailing or phoning coworkers.
- Spend 20 minutes tidying up around the house.
- Stroll around during every American Idol commercial break.
- Never use the moving walkways in airports.

500–1,000
steps

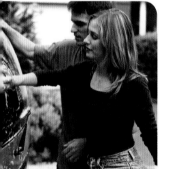

- Walk anyplace that takes less than 5 minutes to reach by car.
- Get up from your desk chair every 90 minutes during the course of an 8-hour day and walk the full perimeter of your business or work area.
- Go for a leisurely 20-minute walk after dinner.
- Spend 15 minutes vacuuming up all the cat hair.
- Do light housework for an hour.
- Spend an hour gardening.
- Wash and wax the car.
- Do an hour of vigorous yoga.
- Stay on your feet and mingle at a cocktail party.
- Park in Goofy 99 and skip the tram at Disney World.

1,000–2,500
steps

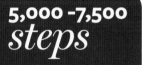

2,500 –5,000 *steps*

- Forget you parked in Goofy 99 and spend 30 minutes hunting for your car at Disney World.
- Take a leisurely 40-minute walk during your lunch hour.
- Grocery-shop for 1 hour.
- Go for a leisurely 1-hour bike ride (pedal strokes are steps, too!)
- Prepare, host, and clean up after a dinner party.
- Walk 30 minutes on a treadmill set at 4 m.p.h.
- Spend a few hours browsing a museum.
- Go bowling.

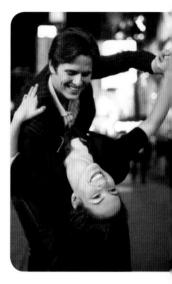

5,000 –7,500 *steps*

- Cut a half-acre lawn with a push mower.
- Spend an afternoon raking up all the leaves you didn't last fall.
- Walk a 5K charity event.
- Spend an afternoon walking around the downtown of a large city.
- Dance the night away.

7,500 –10,000 *steps*

- Stroll back and forth to church on Sunday morning.
- Go golfing using a pull cart.
- Volunteer at a hospital for 8 hours.
- Take the dog for a brisk 60-minute walk.
- Get a part-time job as a waitress.

10,000+ *steps*

- Walk a 10K.
- Spend the day shopping in New York City.
- Walk 90 minutes at a leisurely pace.
- Babysit a four-year-old for 8 hours.

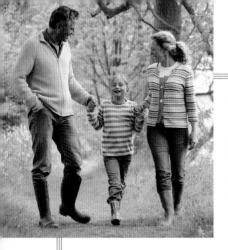

SNEAK IN MORE STEPS

You can put on your gym clothes, sneakers, and pedometer and put in an hour of vigorous walking. Or you can just stride along on a sunny morning alive with birdsong. Or take a lap around the mall before hitting the clearance sales. Or hoof it to the neighborhood mailbox instead of leaving your letter in your own box. Opportunities to walk are endless—and by now you know that the "math" is stunningly simple: The more steps you take, the more calories you'll burn. Here are some ways to sneak more walking into your life and get the most out of every step you take.

Pick a charity and pledge to contribute $1 for every mile you walk.

You'll take pride in the fact that you're walking for a larger cause—and who knows, maybe it will motivate you to go longer and faster. After every walk, mark the amount you owe on a chart, and when you reach $100, send a check. Whoever thought exercise could be tax deductible?

Take your dog with you.

Once Fido gets used to your walks, he'll look forward to them and give you a gentle nudge on the days you try to skip. Don't have a dog? Offer to walk a neighbor's or inquire about walking dogs at a local shelter.

Walk for entertainment once a week.

Instead of padding around your neighborhood, hit the zoo, an art museum, or an upscale shopping mall.

Take the crew for a walk.

This is a perfect way to model good fitness habits for your children. If your children walk too slowly, ask them to ride their bikes or roller-skate alongside you.

Once a week, do your errands on foot.

If you live within a mile of town or even a convenience store, start from your house. If you live out in the middle of nowhere, drive to within a mile of your destination, park, and walk the rest of the way there and back. You'll be surprised how many people you'll meet along the way.

Explore near and far.

Rather than walking the same old tired route day in and day out, use your walks as a way to experience your surroundings. Check out the houses one neighborhood over, walk to a town landmark that you've never been inside, or drive to a park or trailhead to take in the great outdoors.

Walk with a friend.

If she's expecting you, you're more likely to get out of bed instead of burrowing deeper under the covers. At work, look for colleagues to walk with at lunch.

Climb up and down a flight of stairs for 2 minutes.

You'll get your heart rate up in a hurry and build thigh and calf muscles that will propel you faster on your walks.

Burn calories at the kids' ball field.

Instead of taking your folding chair and a crossword puzzle, wear comfortable shoes and take a jaunt around the field.

Walk and talk.

Use your cell phone or cordless and walk around the house as you chat with friends or conduct business. This is a great way to make use of those long times spent on hold with the IRS, or your Internet service provider. The exercise will even help you maintain your mental cool.

Park in Siberia.

Don't fight the hordes for a space near the mall entrance. Instead, park at the perimeter of the lot. You'll save yourself stress and get some more steps in to boot.

Walk in the evening.

After-dinner walks get you away from the television (and the snacks you munch in front of it), keep you from eating too much at dinner, and give you a chance to bump into like-minded neighbors.

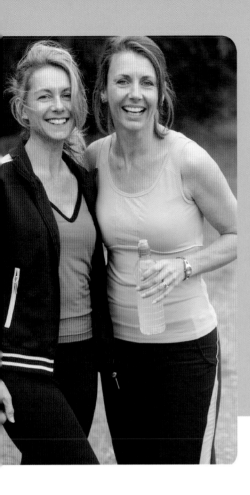

What to *Wear*

Let's be real: All you really need to stride outside is a pair of supportive sneaks and the will to get up and out. But weather, terrain, and safety call for certain clothing items and accessories that can also make exercising more comfortable, productive, and fun.

Aim for Comfort

Fashion isn't king when it comes to walking; comfort is. To get the most out of your walk, you should be completely unconscious of everything you are wearing or carrying when you walk. Out with anything that pinches, pulls, aggravates, or annoys; in with moisture-wicking, friction-reducing, body-supporting, and spirit-boosting clothes, shoes, and accessories. Here are some pointers to keep in mind about what to wear.

On your feet. The most important thing you can do for your walking self is take care of your feet. This means a good-quality shoe that suits your feet and gait, and socks that wick moisture to protect your feet from blisters. See pages 31–32 for more information on how to choose shoes and socks.

WALKING SAFETY 101

Guidelines for staying safe wherever and whenever you walk are simple:

• Always carry your ID in your pocket.

• Program your ICE (In Case of Emergency) contact info into your cell phone.

• Wear a reflective vest or armbands when you walk in low light, morning or evening, or in inclement weather.

• Stay on familiar public paths and roadways when walking alone.

• Walk with a partner when you're in an unfamiliar place.

On your legs. Shorts, a skirt, or pants (depending on temperature) that are light-weight, breathable, and don't pinch or bind anywhere is best. So is a zippered pocket for your ID, keys, or cash.

On top. A lightweight, breathable tank or a short- or long-sleeved tee will suit warm or moderate temperatures. Add a hoodie and/or a vest for cooler weather and you also get the flexibility of layering.

On your head. A visor or baseball-style cap made of a lightweight, ventilated fabric will keep you cool and provide UV protection. At the least, you should wear sun-glasses that provide 100 percent UV protection and block the sun and wind, which is especially important if you wear contacts. Look for sports shades, which are designed to stay put even when you work up a sweat.

In your hands. Nothing. It's best to keep both hands free so your arms are able to move naturally. Clip your pedometer to your waist, along with your music player or cell phone, if carrying either or both. Clip a BPA-free refillable water bottle to your waist, too. And if you're carrying all of the above gadgets, consider a lightweight waist pack with zippered pockets and a hook that can accommodate your water bottle.

That's it. There are countless high-end sports stores, catalogs, and websites that would be happy to sell you a bunch of pricey walking clothes and gadgetry if that's how you roll, but really, the items listed above are all you need to get your Walk It Off program in gear.

Sneaker Features That Will Move You

Barefoot marathon runners aside, most of us need shoes to cushion our paws as we put miles of pavement behind us. But if you're walking in a running shoe, you're doing your feet a disservice. You wouldn't wear downhill skis to cross-country ski, would you?

The features that you can't see are the most important. "Walking shoes are meant to flex near the front of the shoe, allowing a full heel-to-toe rolling range of motion," explains Douglas Richie, DPM, a podiatrist based in Seal Beach, California.

Wondering if your shoes are fit for the job? Try this simple test: Hold one shoe in both hands and try to twist it. "It should resist twisting," says Dr. Richie. Now take the toe end of the shoe and bend it back slightly. This should be fairly easy to do. The twist and flex tests are important, Dr. Richie adds, because "most so-called walking shoes are too stiff and not designed for true fitness walking."

Well-designed walking shoes will provide ample cushioning in the heel and fore-foot to absorb shock and keep your feet stable as you move from heel to toe. Before you go out and buy a new pair of walkers, though, identify which kind of feet you have; this will determine what shoe you should be wearing. Work with an experienced sports-shoe salesperson to be sure you're getting the best shoe for your particular needs—and budget.

For Walkers Who Pronate or Supinate

If your feet tend to pronate (collapse inward) or supinate (roll outward), you need to wear walking shoes that help you compensate for these tendencies. How do you know which you are? Check out the soles of your current sneakers. If the soles are worn along the outside edges of the forefoot and heel, you're a supinator. If they're worn along the inside edges, you're a pronator. Be sure to let the shoe salesperson know which you are; better yet, bring along your old sneakers so she can assess for herself what your particular issues are. You will likely be pointed to a shoe with motion-control features, including an insole that promotes a smooth heel-to-toe stride, as well as a well-defined arch for those who need a lift. Cushioning in the heel boosts rebound and reduces foot fatigue.

For Walkers with "Neutral" Feet

Neutral feet are those that don't tend to roll inward or outward. When you try on sneakers, remember that they should feel comfortable right away, with no break-in period. Look for shoes with adequate support, and shock-absorbant cushioning that protects during the heel-strike part of each step. Because you don't need a shoe that corrects your gait, you have the most flexibility regarding the material the upper part of your shoe is made of—lightweight mesh or sturdier leather. It's up to you.

For Walkers with Narrow or Wide Feet

If you have wide or narrow feet, your shoes should feature supportive insoles and shock-absorbant cushioned outsoles that help you maintain a straightforward, smooth stride.

SHOES THAT ROCK ON—OR DO THEY?

People looking to get extra exercise with each step—or to make a fashion statement—are flocking to shoes with convex soles that allow them to rock back and forth. Made popular by the brand MBT (Masai Barefoot Technology), they're designed to stretch leg muscles and make your legs, hips, and glutes work harder than they do in regular athletic shoes. Because they're unsteady, they're said to recruit core muscles to help you balance. So do they work?

"The soles do put a greater load on the calf and hamstring muscles, which presumably could strengthen them," says Dr. Richie. There isn't proof of that yet, but in studies sponsored by the manufacturers, the shoes have improved posture and reduced joint stress in people who wear them.

"If you have a condition like neuropathy, diabetes, arthritis, or muscle weakness around the ankles, the shoes might make walking more comfortable," concludes Dr. Richie. MBTs can be expensive, though other brands, including Skechers Shape-ups, are cheaper. Manufacturers recommend wearing them only for short periods until you get used to them.

6 WAYS TO ACE YOUR LACING

You probably thought you'd mastered the art of tying your shoes in kindergarten. But with these lacing tricks, you can tailor the fit of your walking shoe to the shape of your foot to help prevent and relieve foot problems.

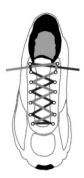

PROBLEM: Slipping heel

SOLUTION: Create a lace lock

Starting at the toe end, lace in the traditional crisscross pattern, stopping at the second-to-last eyelet. Thread into the top eyelet on the side each lace has just exited. This creates a small loop. Thread each lace through the loop on the opposite side to create a "locked" fit.

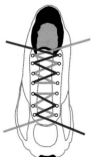

PROBLEM: Narrow heel with wide forefoot

SOLUTION: Use two short laces

With one short shoelace, start at the middle of the shoe and lace in a normal crisscross pattern, ending

at the toe end. Tie. Use the second lace on the top half, and lace the shoe more tightly, tying at the top. If your heel slips, finish with a lace lock.

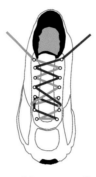

PROBLEM: Narrow foot

SOLUTION: Lock laces halfway

Starting at the toe end, lace in a crisscross pattern, stopping at the second or third eyelet, depending on where your foot becomes narrow (and on how many eyelets your shoe has). Thread each lace through the next eyelet on the side it has just exited, making a small loop. Thread the end of the opposite lace through each loop and pull to create a lock. Continue crisscrossing.

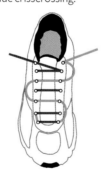

PROBLEM: High arch

SOLUTION: Create an "S" shape

Start at the toe end of the right shoe and thread the lace down through the first set of eyelets. Thread the right-hand end up through the next

eyelet on the same side, then across and down through the eyelet on the other side. Now thread it up the same side again, skipping an eyelet. Take it across, then repeat. Cross at the top. Repeat with the other lace.

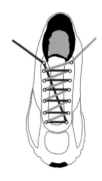

PROBLEM: Toe pain

SOLUTION: Elevate the laces

Thread from the top right-hand eyelet through to the bottom left, leaving enough lace at the top to tie. Crisscross from the bottom and tie.

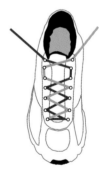

PROBLEM: Pain on top of feet

SOLUTION: Leave a space

Lace up the bottom four eyelets in the standard crisscross pattern. Next, thread the laces straight up through the eyelets until you reach the top two eyelets. Crisscross again and tie.

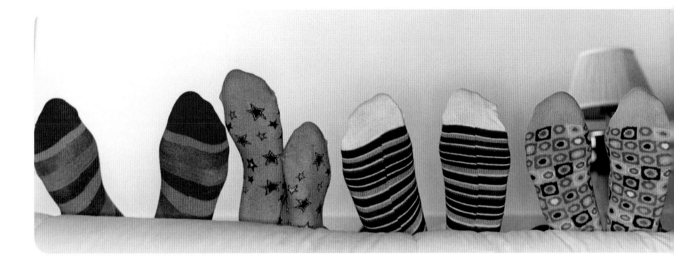

Boost Your Socks Appeal

It's amazing that the most dedicated walker can be fussy about choosing the right shoe but throw on any old pair of socks before hitting the road. The wrong pair of socks can ruin a perfectly good walk, according to Karen Langone, a podiatrist in Southampton, New York, and president of the American Academy of Podiatric Sports Medicine.

She's referring, of course, to every walker's enemy number one: blisters. "If you're not walking in a moisture-managing sock and your feet get sweaty, chafing and blisters are inevitable," she contends. So take a pass on those $5 six-packs of cotton sport socks you see at the mega stores. Pure cotton soaks up and retains moisture, making it ideal for towels but terrible for toes.

Still, are pricey-by-comparison athletic socks made from blends of synthetic and natural fibers (including wool, silk, and yes, cotton) worth the price tag? We say yes. Read on and you'll see why.

Keep your fibers straight.

Much of the research devoted to athletic "hosiery" during the last couple of decades originated in the military. That's because blisters are the bane of soldiers everywhere. Textile companies were challenged to develop fabrics that were quick drying, comfortable, and durable, and they have mostly succeeded. Today walkers and runners, skiers and snowboarders, cyclists and tennis players benefit from the military-driven R&D that brought us "hydrophilic" fibers, which absorb moisture and wick that moisture off the skin to the outer surface of the sock, where it can more easily evaporate. And of course, makers have come up with lots of ways to make socks thicker or thinner, warmer or cooler. Here are some of the most popular and effective athletic-sock fibers now available:

CoolMax is a synthetic fiber engineered to quickly transport perspiration away from the skin and to the surface of the sock. CoolMax is breathable even when wet and helps regulate temperature and keep feet dry.

SOCKS MATTER. TO AVOID BLISTERS, WEAR SOCKS MADE OF HYDROPHILIC FIBERS, WHICH WICK MOISTURE AWAY FROM THE SKIN.

MAKE THEM LAST

A good pair of socks, worn once a week, should last at least two years—much longer than the cotton athletic socks of the past. That's in large part because today's socks are usually reinforced in the high-wear areas like toes and heels.

According to sock manufacturer Kris Dahlgren, the number one reason that athletic socks develop holes early in their lives is because they snag on long, jagged toenails. "Keep your toenails trimmed and your socks will last longer," she says. If you do develop a hole or notice a thin spot, repair it by stitching well beyond the hole. Then try on the sock. If you can feel the repaired area rubbing against your skin, it's probably time to turn it into a pull toy for Fido.

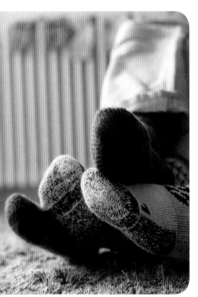

Polypropylene is a lightweight synthetic fiber that is also excellent at wicking moisture.

Microfiber acrylics tend to be "low bulk" fibers (meaning they're thin) that are super soft and moisture wicking.

Merino and alpaca wools are itchless because their fibers are long and silky. Wool is the most hydrophilic natural fiber and is able to absorb as much as 30 percent of its weight in moisture without feeling wet. When combined with synthetic fibers, such as CoolMax or polypropylene, the wool absorbs moisture and the synthetic fibers move it away from the skin.

Lycra and Spandex provide stretch and memory fit in athletic socks. It's the reason that a sock heel still has a "cup" even after repeated wearings.

Thermolite provides warmth and comfort without weight, even when it's wet. It has hollow fibers that trap air for insulation, but also speed moisture away from the skin. Thermolite also dries 20 percent faster than other insulating fabrics and 50 percent faster than cotton.

Silver fibers go by various trade names, such as X-STATIC or SmartSilver, but they all act as antimicrobials, meaning they inhibit the growth of fungi and bacteria. This makes them popular among people who are prone to foot odor and infections.

Bamboo and Cocona are two new "green" fibers that have taken the athletic sock market by storm. Cocona is made from coconut shells; sock manufacturers like it because it's super soft, quick drying, and odor absorbing. Bamboo has similar properties and feels like silk.

Sock seasons

When it's warm out, look for socks with an inner layer of synthetic fiber, such as CoolMax or polypropylene, to transfer moisture away from the skin and keep your feet dry.

During winter, choose fabrics that provide insulation from the cold but still release moisture. Wool is the best natural fiber for warmth. Even when wet, wool is warm because its fibers trap air, providing insulation. Just remember that wool blends rather than pure wool are best for athletic pursuits because the synthetic fibers pull moisture away from the skin.

Fit matters

The fit of the socks you exercise in matters as much as the fit of your shoes. Socks should fit the length and width of your feet snugly without being tight. "Overly tight socks can bind your toes and feel really uncomfortable," says Dr. Langone. Loose ones can bunch up in your shoes, causing chafing and blisters. For walking, you want socks that have flat-knit toe seams so there's no rubbing or bulkiness. The heels should be flexible, with a "Y" heel seam or a heel pocket, so the sock doesn't slide around or slip down.

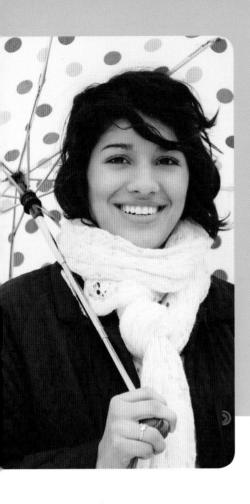

"*Weather*" to Walk

Just about any weather is walking weather, as long as you're appropriately dressed for comfort and safety. A good rule of thumb is if temperature, visibility, and surfaces are safe enough for riding a bicycle, you're good to go for a walk. Staying dry on a wet day, keeping warm on a cold day, and not getting too overheated on a hot day is about all you need to worry about.

When It's Wet

If you have waterproof shoes and outer clothing, you can look forward to singing—and walking—in the rain. If you don't, you might want to consider hitting the mall or the treadmill instead of venturing outside.

For a rainy day walker, waterproof shoes are a must. They can be expensive, but because keeping your feet dry is an absolute requirement, it's worth it. Look for waterproof outer materials and/or a Gore-Tex lining. Wear good-quality moisture-wicking (not cotton) socks, too.

Wear a hooded waterproof rain jacket or slicker (depending on the temperature). Plastic ponchos are only good for when you're caught in the rain; they're impractical for regular use because they're not really waterproof and the wind easily has its way with them. A baseball cap worn under the hood of your jacket can add a little protection from the rain if the wind isn't a factor. And waterproof rain pants are a good investment if you're an avid rainy day walker.

Waiting for a bus? Grab that umbrella. Going for a walk? Not such a good idea. Umbrellas can be awkward to maneuver in heavy rain or wind. They can also make it difficult for you to be seen or to react quickly in a pinch. If walking is your objective, try to do without the umbrella.

Safety is a prime consideration when walking in the rain. A driver's visibility is already impaired due to the weather, so wear a vest, armband, or hat with a reflective feature to ensure you can be seen at a safe distance.

When It's Cold

THE FIRST RULE OF PREPARING TO WALK IN THE COLD IS TO DRESS IN LAYERS.

The first rule of preparing to walk in the cold is to dress in layers. Your base layer (silk or synthetic, not cotton) should wick sweat away from your body to keep your skin dry. Next comes an insulating layer of wool or fleece you can adjust at the neck and wrists or shed as you warm up. Your loose-fitting outer layer should be wind- and waterproof.

In extreme cold, hoods and draw cords at the neck, waist, wrists, and ankles of your outerwear will help keep the draft out. To keep essential body heat from escaping, a hat is a must; a fleece cap with earflaps is ideal. A scarf does double duty, keeping the neck warm and wrapping around the face to protect against the wind, as necessary. Finish with wind- and waterproof mittens, which keep your hands warmer than gloves.

Wear wool or multilayer socks, waterproof hiking shoes, and consider adding traction boosters to your shoes to keep you steady on unexpected slippery surfaces. Drink water to stay hydrated, just as you would on the hottest day of the year. And finally, apply lip protector and sunscreen to any exposed skin.

When It's Hot

If you don't mind the heat (and some people do), there's nothing wrong with walking in it. You just need to pay attention to hydration, sun exposure, and wearing clothes, shoes, and other gear that does no harm on a hot day.

First rule of hot-weather walking is to plan for full hydration. If your water supply is about to run out, it's time to head home. Remember, your body is actually thirsty about 20 minutes before your brain tells you so. Drink a large glass of water before you leave for your walk, then another 8 ounces every mile or so as you go.

Protect yourself from sun exposure by applying the highest UV protection sunscreen all over your body, not just where the skin is openly exposed. The sun's UV rays can penetrate most fabrics, so it's best to apply before dressing to go outdoors. And wear a visor or breathable hat and sunglasses to protect your face and eyes from UV rays and harsh sun glare.

Wear a breathable, moisture-wicking top and shorts. Wear bicycle-style shorts if your thighs tend to chafe. You might also apply anti-chafing cream at your underarms or thighs. Finally, wear your best-quality moisture-wicking socks and well-fitting broken-in shoes to prevent blisters.

And the most important rule to remember when out and about on a hot day is to know when enough's enough. If you push yourself too hard, you can increase chances of heat sickness. Pay attention to signs of dehydration, including fatigue, dizziness, stomachache, headache, and dry mouth. Signs of extreme loss of body salts include nausea, dizziness, cramps, headache, confusion, and trouble speaking. If this happens, get out of the sun and replenish your electrolytes with a sports drink. And consider taking it easy until that cold front arrives!

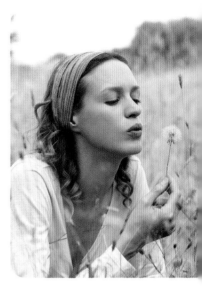

WHEN *NOT* TO WALK

When wondering whether to walk or not, the weather should rarely hold you back. If, however, you find yourself feeling off, it's wise to take the day off, too. Stay off your feet—and check in with your doctor—if you've got:

- A lingering cold, the flu, or a fever
- More fatigue than usual
- A swollen or painful muscle or joint
- A new or undiagnosed symptom
- Chest pain or an irregular, rapid, or fluttery heartbeat
- Shortness of breath

When It's Allergy Season

Neither rain, nor snow, nor dark of night can keep you from your walk. Allergies, though, can really throw a monkey wrench into your walking plans. We want to be outside and moving, enjoying the return of flowers, grass, leaves, and warmth in the spring. But doing that without sneezing, coughing, or getting congested? Not so easy.

Allergies can't be cured. But by knowing how they work and actively managing the condition, there's absolutely no reason for allergies to keep you from lacing up.

Know thy enemy

In simplest terms allergies occur when your body encounters non-dangerous items and tags them as dangerous. The vast majority of allergens are airborne and include dust, pollen, mold, and pet dander. When they enter your body, your immune system responds by going on the offensive.

Symptoms of seasonal allergies are pretty common: sneezing; a clear, runny nose; itchy or dry eyes; headache; stuffy, inflamed sinuses. Colds and allergies are often mistaken for each other, but colds come on more slowly. Allergies come on quickly, and usually at the same time each year or after a long time outside during allergy season.

Of all the allergens, pollen—the microscopic round or oval grains that plants use in lieu of sex to reproduce—is the one responsible for the misery of tens of millions of Americans. Among North American plants, weeds are the most prolific springtime producers of allergenic pollen, with ragweed the major culprit; others include sagebrush, redroot pigweed, lamb's-quarters, Russian thistle (tumbleweed), and English plantain. A single ragweed plant can generate a million grains a day.

How to fight back

New technologies allow us to quickly and accurately determine how many grains of a specific pollen or mold are found in a set volume of air (usually a cubic meter) over 24 hours. This information, known as the pollen count, is extremely useful to people with allergies, since it tells them if they are more or less likely to have allergic reactions if they stay outside. Daily data about local pollen count is available online, included in most local weather forecasts, and can even be downloaded to your smart phone.

The most common allergy medicines are antihistamines. These do exactly what their name says: They counteract the effects of histamine, the inflammatory chemical released by your body during an allergic reaction. In effect, antihistamines shut down an allergic reaction by turning off your immune system's response.

Other common allergy medicines include decongestants to unclog your nose and sinuses, and anticholinergic sprays, prescription medicine that shuts down mucous production. For people who suffer from severe reactions, doctors prescribe emergency medications, like epinephrine.

First, get an accurate diagnosis of what causes your allergies; it's so much easier to avoid a few specific allergens than to worry about everything that's out there. If the allergens are within your house, get cleaning! If your allergies are due to outdoor pollens or molds, talk to your doctor about whether it makes sense for you to take antihistamines prior to an outdoor walk. Also pay close attention to pollen counts and their cycles. Most plants release pollen early in the morning, and they are often most prevalent in the air around noon, making evening the best time to walk.

Finally, study up on what makes your immune system healthiest (Pssst! The answer is plenty of fresh produce, exercise, and effective stress management), and follow through. Research clearly shows that having a weak immune system increases your chances of allergic reactions or asthma attacks.

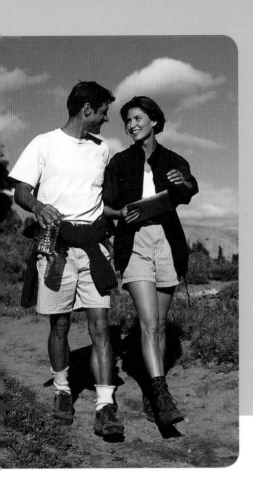

Where to Walk

The beauty of walking is that you can do it anywhere. Really. Outdoors, indoors, on the street, on the track, on the treadmill—there's no limit to the places you can get the job done. There are some natural advantages of some venues over others, but they've all got their own specific benefits.

Take It Outside

Why walk outdoors? There are about a million reasons, but for starters, do it for the fresh air, the full engagement of your senses, its ability to improve your mood, and the exposure to natural sunlight, the body's best source of vitamin D. Add to that the physical benefits, such as improving your balance and strengthening your muscles with every step up and down a curb or hill. Streets, sidewalks, and natural paths offer constant challenge, causing you to compensate for uneven terrain, sudden obstacles, and occasional stops and starts. That's why walking outside absolutely offers the best variety of conditions, which helps deliver an effective fat-burning workout.

Soft surfaces, like dirt, sand, or grass, are easier on your joints than street asphalt or cement sidewalks. And because soft surfaces have some give, they also force you to work a little harder and use more energy (and burn more calories). For example, walking on packed sand burns 50 percent more calories than walking at the same pace on a sidewalk.

Sidewalks and streets generally offer a more consistent surface than a natural path, although they certainly present their own challenges. There's a reason they sometimes call walking "pounding the pavement!" Asphalt and sidewalk surfaces can be unforgiving, which is why wearing good walking shoes is so important. There's also the unfortunate reality of potholes, broken curbs and sidewalks, and other evidence of poorly maintained streets that can make safe walking a challenge. This just means you need to pay attention while you walk; don't get so caught up in your iPod revelry that you don't see the asphalt crater that's about to swallow you whole! Seriously, if you don't watch where you walk, you could easily end up with skinned knees and elbows or a twisted ankle.

If you don't want to worry about the particular challenges natural paths, streets, and sidewalks present, a track can be an excellent outdoor alternative. The material from which most tracks are constructed is designed to provide a perfectly consistent and firm but shock-absorbent surface, which makes a track a natural choice for beginners and veterans alike, as well as someone who is prone to shin splints or recovering from an injury. You don't need to worry about curbs or crosswalks on a track, but without any incline, you need to be sure to mix up your pace in order to get your heart rate up and pumping.

DON'T HOLD THE HANDRAILS ON A TREADMILL. MOVING YOUR ARMS BURNS CALORIES AND IT'S BETTER FOR YOUR POSTURE.

Opting for Inner Peace

For someone with arthritis or a similar chronic condition, the upside of walking outside—the uneven terrain, the regular obstacles, the stops and starts—is actually a downside. One wrong step can aggravate the condition and set you back on your weight-loss goal.

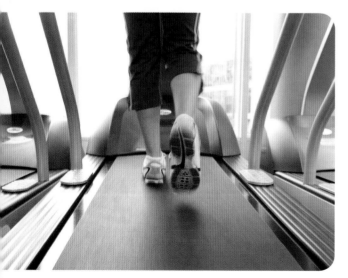

The treadmill. As mentioned earlier, the track is a great place for folks who need a safe, consistent surface. So is a treadmill. Although the moving tread propelling you and the lack of wind resistance is likely to decrease the amount of calories you burn compared to walking outdoors, you can make up for this by setting the treadmill at a slight incline (1%) at all times. And be sure to avoid holding the handrails; moving your arms burns more calories, and it's better for your posture, too.

For the best workout, be sure to mix it up. While you work a greater variety of muscles when walking outside, especially because of the uphills *and* the downhills, the treadmill still offers the ability to increase and decrease your pace and to add inclines that can provide a significant workout.

TREADMILL TRAINING

Your treadmill walks don't need to be boring. There are terrific MP3 programs that combine energetic music, audio coaching, and prompts to go faster or increase your incline for short periods to add challenge to your workout. Think of those spin class instructors calling out instructions and encouragement to the riders, who are all pedaling madly to the pulsing music. That's what's happening in your ears when you walk with one of these programs on your MP3.

There are also video treadmill programs you can pop into your DVD; one type is a visual demonstration of different workouts you can do on your treadmill, and the other is simply for the atmosphere, with scenes from beautiful beaches, forests, and mountains all over the world, filmed from a walker's perspective. If you have got a good imagination, you could be walking at sunset on a beach in Hawaii!

The mall. It goes without saying, of course, that when snow, rain, sleet, and hail threaten to keep you from your walk, the treadmill saves the day. But so can the mall. Often open early to accommodate walkers, malls are a great, safe place to walk alone or in groups, with the added benefit of access to restrooms and drinking water. It not only provides the consistent surface of a track but also a comfortable climate, no matter what the season. If you live in Miami in the summer or Minnesota in the winter, the mall may be just the place to get in your 10,000 steps.

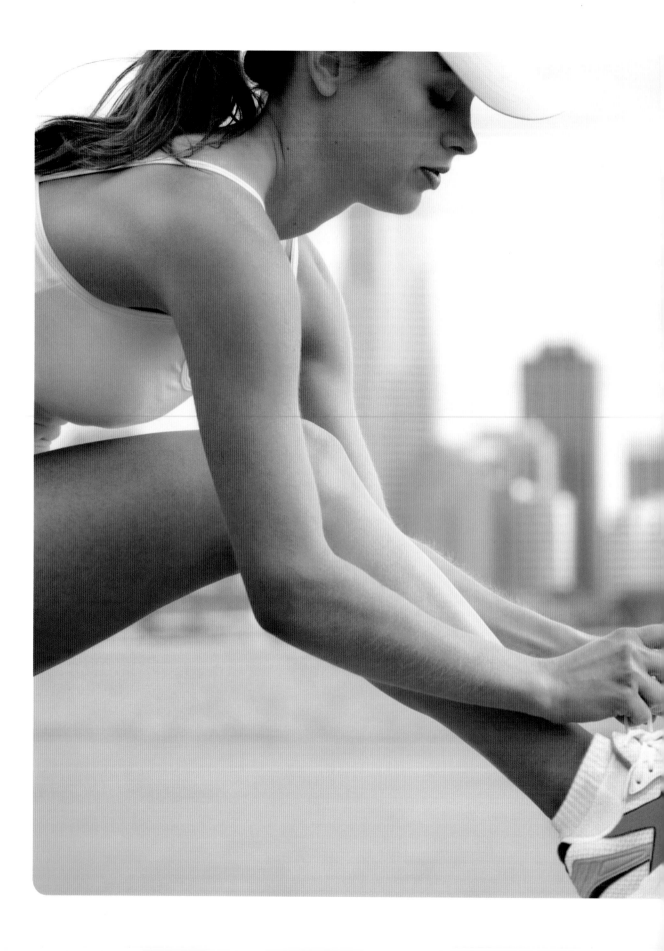

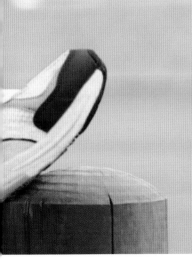

Let's Take
a Walk

THE BEST PART OF WALKING is that you can start it right here, right now, before you turn another page. It's that easy. If you decide to pursue walking as the fitness component of your weight-loss plan, it's always a good idea to mention this to your doctor, who may have specific advice for you based on your medical history. And whether you turn into a fierce fitness walker or remain a blissful daydreamy stroller, remember not to overdo it, especially when you're just getting started.

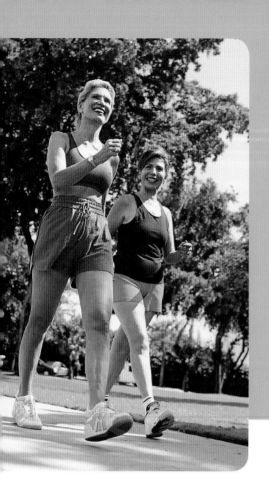

Get Started on Your Journey

If the last exercise you remember doing was in high school gym class, ease into walking gradually, starting with 15 minutes at a time and working up to 20- and 30-minute walks. Pay attention to your heart rate and stop if you feel discomfort anywhere in your body. It takes almost no time for your body to adapt to walking—which it knows how to do naturally, after all!—and you will be comfortable handling 30-, 45-, and even 60-minute walks before you know it.

At first, though, focus on shorter walks that will allow you to become familiar with how your body feels when you walk at varying paces. Pay attention, too, to the way you carry your body when you walk. It's important to walk correctly—with good posture, balanced movement, and a clean gait—in order to get the most bang for your exercise buck and, of course, to help avoid injury.

Tracking Your Heart Rate

To track your heart rate during your walks, invest in a heart-rate monitor. Good brands start at about $60. With many models you can input your age and your resting and maximum heart rates so the device automatically calculates your heart-rate status. (To calculate your resting heart rate, check your pulse when you first wake up. Count the number of heartbeats in 30 seconds, then multiply by 2.)

Don't have a heart-rate monitor? You can still track your heart rate. All you need is a watch with a second hand. Simply place the tips of your first two fingers on your inner wrist or on your lower neck on either side of your windpipe. Press lightly until you feel your pulse. Count the number of pulses over 6 seconds, then multiply that number by 10 to get a rough estimate of your heart rate.

If you don't want to bother with a monitor or taking your pulse, see below for a sense of how hard you'll need to work to get your heart rate into the various target zones.

Guesstimate

No heart rate monitor? No problem! It's easy to guess how fast your heart is pumping by observing how much—or how little—you're able to speak while walking. Here's how, in a nutshell.

- *50 to 60 percent of your max:*

Brisk walking. You can carry on a conversation, though you might breathe a little hard.

- *60 to 70 percent of your max:*

Very fast walking. You can speak only in short sentences.

- *70 to 80 percent of your max:*

Walking as fast as you can. You can utter only a few words.

- *80 to 85 percent of your max:*

Walking as fast as you can up a big hill, pumping your arms aggressively. Speaking is nearly impossible.

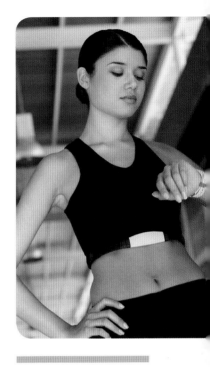

EVENTUALLY YOU'LL DEVELOP A NATURAL SENSE OF YOUR HEART-RATE RANGE AT VARIOUS LEVELS OF EXERTION. UNTIL THEN, USE A HEART MONITOR OR A WATCH WITH A SECOND HAND TO DETERMINE YOUR HEART RATE.

WHAT'S YOUR MAX?

To calculate your maximum heart rate, simply subtract your age from 220.

220 _____ – _____ =

(your maximum   (your age
heart rate)   in years)

If you are 40 years old, for example, your maximum heart rate is 180 beats per minute. If you want to work out at 50 percent of your maximum, multiply your maximum by 0.5

THE MECHANICS OF WALKING

While there may be variables to take into account when you walk, such as speed or terrain, the only thing you really need to do when you walk is to use good form. It will make walking feel easier and help prevent injuries, too. Do it like this:

HEAD
Imagine a string attached to the top of your head pulling your crown toward the sky.

SHOULDERS
Keep your shoulders relaxed, down, and slightly back.

ARMS
Keep your elbows bent at about 90-degree angles. Pump them forward and back; they shouldn't cross in front of your body.

BACK
Stand up straight, not hunched forward.

CHEST
Keep your breastbone lifted and shining forward. Yoga practitioners call this area your "heart light."

LEGS
Maintain a natural stride length; it should not feel strained. Longer isn't better.

FEET
Land first on your heel, then roll forward across the ball of your foot and push off with your toes.

The 5 Biggest Walking Missteps

We know what you're thinking: How can anyone screw up at walking? That's like botching up breathing or sleeping. Well, it's actually more common than you might think (and, surprisingly, chewing gum has nothing to do with it). Many new walkers get bored, discouraged, injured, or just aren't having as much fun as they should because they're unwittingly doing some things wrong. Here are five frequent mistakes that could be hurting you or holding you back.

Wearing worn-out shoes

The cushioning properties of even the best sports shoes break down with use. This can lead to discomfort and eventually injury, especially if you're overweight. There's no mystery to knowing when it's time for a new shoe; if you see worn areas on the soles, it's time to get yourself a new pair. To get the best fit, shop in the afternoon when your feet are biggest, wear the socks you'll be walking in, make sure there's a little space between your big toe and the end of the shoe, and walk around the store to be sure the heel doesn't slip.

Walking without warming up

Most people don't think of walking as a strenuous activity, but if you spend most of your day sitting at a desk, then you're essentially asking your body to spring out of the blocks. Before you start really hoofing it, you need to elevate your core body temperature, get the blood and oxygen flowing to the muscles, and lubricate your joints. Take 3 minutes to do slow ankle, hip, and arm circles (not all at once!) and you'll be ready to roll.

WARM IT UP

Contrary to what fitness experts used to believe, a warm-up should not consist of heavy or strenuous stretching. This could actually tire out your muscles and cause injury. Save the serious stretching for your cool-down (see chapter 3, "Get Fit to Walk It Off," for tips on stretching, strength training, and boosting your flexibility). To warm up before a walk, an easy 5-minute stroll or 5 minutes of gentle stretching is all you need to increase the temperature and blood flow in the muscles you use most when walking, which will make your experience more comfortable and enjoyable. Here are some you could try:

Ankle circles. Standing, lift one foot off the floor, point the toe, and rotate your ankle 10 times in one direction, then 10 times in the other. Repeat on the other side.

Toe points. Standing, lift one foot off the floor, point the toe, and hold for 5 seconds. Now flex the same foot and hold for 5 seconds. Do this 5 times for each foot.

Quad stretch. Standing, bend one leg at the knee and reach behind you to grasp your foot or ankle. Gently pull your foot to stretch the front of the thigh, holding for up to 10 seconds. Repeat on the other side.

Overhead stretch. Standing with feet hip-width apart, reach your hands up over your head, palms facing forward with your arms forming a V. Gently move your hands back, as if someone is pushing against them, and hold for up to 10 seconds. Next, bend one elbow and drop your hand to touch your back, holding for 5 seconds. Relax the first arm and repeat with the other.

Using poor technique

Overstriding, foot-slapping, head-hanging, chicken-winging, arm-flinging—these are just a few of the common flaws that can lead to inefficiency and injury. When walking, remember to square up your posture, swing your arms bent at 90 degrees close to your body, push off evenly (heel to midfoot to toes) with every step, and maintain an even stride, no matter how fast or slow you're walking. Better yet, ask a friend to videotape you walking. Evaluate your posture, arm swing, step, and stride. You'll immediately see what you need to correct.

Not stretching afterward

Most new walkers forego cooldowns. But just as muscles and tendons need to ease into an activity, they also need to ease out. Otherwise, they can tighten and cramp. The older you get, the more important it is to stretch after being active. Take 3 minutes to do slow standing lunges, gentle bent-waist forward stretches with slightly flexed knees, and overhead bent arm stretches, as if you're scratching the top of your back.

Not setting specific goals

As with everything else in life, if your goals aren't clear, realistic, and measurable, it's unlikely you'll reach them. The simple solution is to measure your success in steps. Use a pedometer all day, every day, both when you're walking for exercise and just moving through your day. Determine how many steps you're taking without trying, then find ways to add 10 to 20 percent each week until you reach 10,000 steps a day. Your body will continue to reset itself to its increased capacity and will actually crave the benefits this amount of movement provides.

Three Walks to Get the Ball Rolling

No one expects you to walk out the door and make it to the top of Mt. Kilimanjaro and back on your first walk. In fact, no matter how enthusiastic you're feeling about starting your walking program, if you haven't exercised for a long time, ease into walking with short 15-, 20-, then 25-minute walks that will help your body acclimate to the activity.

An added bonus? It's easy to work short walks into a busy schedule. Squeeze in four 15-minute jaunts and you've walked for an hour! Here are three simple walking programs to get you started on the walking-for-weight-loss journey.

Walk It Off PLAYLIST

R&B/Soul

"Crazy In Love,"
Beyoncé

"Proud Mary,"
Tina Turner

"Forget You,"
Cee Lo Green

"I Feel Good,"
James Brown

"Knock You Down,"
Keri Hilson, Kanye West,
Ne-Yo

"Kiss"
(Extended version),
Prince

"Fallin',"
Alicia Keys

"Freeway of Love,"
Aretha Franklin

"You Know I'm No Good,"
Amy Winehouse with
Ghostface Killah

"Ain't No Mountain
High Enough,"
Marvin Gaye and
Tammi Terrell

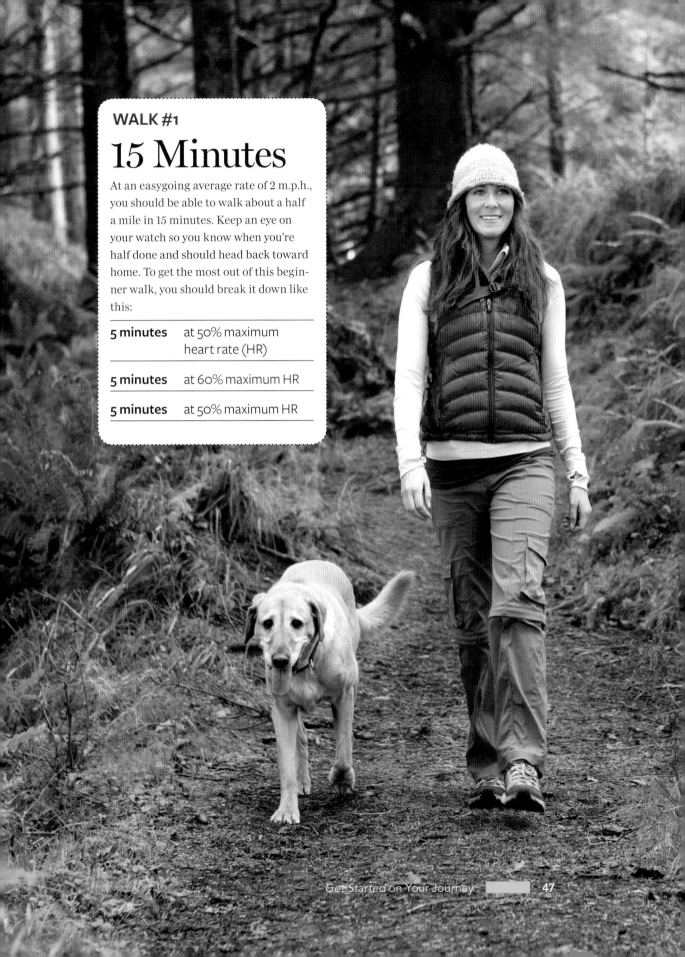

WALK #1

15 Minutes

At an easygoing average rate of 2 m.p.h., you should be able to walk about a half a mile in 15 minutes. Keep an eye on your watch so you know when you're half done and should head back toward home. To get the most out of this beginner walk, you should break it down like this:

5 minutes	at 50% maximum heart rate (HR)
5 minutes	at 60% maximum HR
5 minutes	at 50% maximum HR

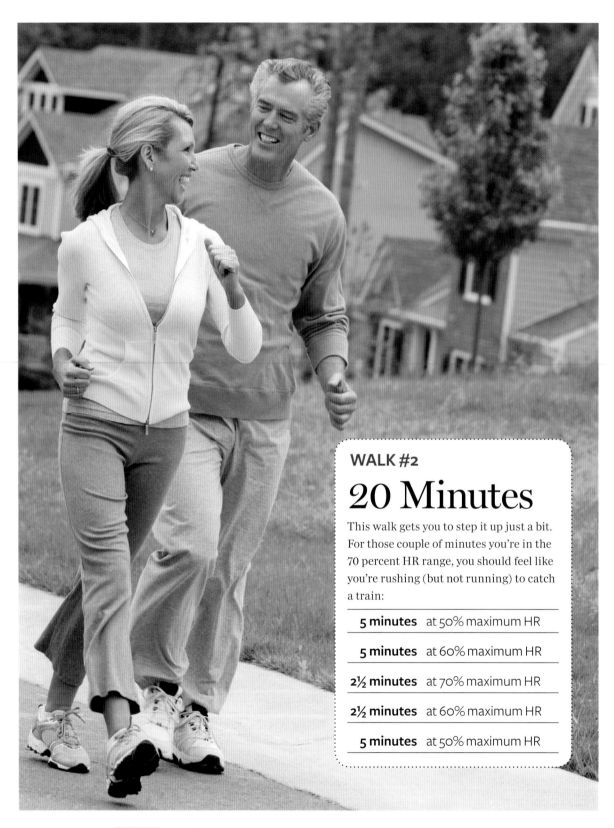

WALK #2

20 Minutes

This walk gets you to step it up just a bit. For those couple of minutes you're in the 70 percent HR range, you should feel like you're rushing (but not running) to catch a train:

5 minutes	at 50% maximum HR
5 minutes	at 60% maximum HR
2½ minutes	at 70% maximum HR
2½ minutes	at 60% maximum HR
5 minutes	at 50% maximum HR

WALK #3

25 minutes

This walk features short interval bursts to boost your heart rate and calorie burning.

5 minutes	at 50% maximum HR
5 minutes	at 60% maximum HR
2½ minutes	at 70% maximum HR
2½ minutes	at 60% maximum HR
2½ minutes	at 70% maximum HR
2½ minutes	at 60% maximum HR
5 minutes	at 50% maximum HR

Try to identify three or four handy half-mile to 1-mile routes you might take for these short walks. How many city blocks would it take on your lunch hour? Two to four laps at the high school track or the mall would do the trick, too.

Having a few go-to distance-measured routes will help you plan your walks and stick to your program.

WALK WITH PURPOSE

We've established that the best way to think about walking is to consider it a natural, seamlessly integrated part of your day-to-day life rather than as a formal exercise regime. One way to achieve this mindset is to build habits and routines where walking goes hand in hand with other activities you care about. Here are a dozen delightful things you can do while putting one foot in front of the other.

Window-shop.

Map a route that weaves through the downtown shopping district, or drive to the nearest mall and do a few laps. Consider it a reconnaissance mission that will save you shopping time later. But make sure to leave your purse and credit cards behind so you aren't tempted to stop, spend, and otherwise interrupt your workout.

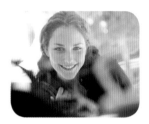

Bird-watch.

Some great new mobile phone apps can help you identify your feathered friends. These include iBird Explorer Plus, Audubon Birds, and National Geographic Hand-Held Birds. Peruse your phone's app store for one that fits your needs and budget; iBird Plus, for instance, even has audioclips of bird songs and calls so you can chirp back.

Reconnect.

Walking not only opens our hearts to nature but also to each other. Many people find it easier to broach difficult subjects and talk honestly while walking, plus people tend to listen better because of fewer distractions. If you need to hash out an issue with your mate, break through to your mystery teen, or just reconnect with a friend, try doing so while walking.

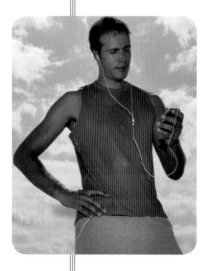

Read.

If you love to curl up with a good book but rarely have the luxury, visit audible.com, download a classic or current bestseller, and listen on your iPod or mobile phone as you walk. Your local library also has audiobooks in CD and cassette formats for lending.

Meditate.

Some people naturally find it easier to meditate while walking than sitting. There's something about the rhythmic, repetitive action of putting one foot in front of the other that fosters inner peace. To experience it, adopt an easy, consistent pace and become aware of your heel and then your mid-foot and finally your toes hitting the ground on each forward step. Synchronize your breath. Forget. You'll know you've hit the sweet spot when the minutes pass like seconds and you finish even more refreshed than when you started.

Learn a language.

If you've ever struggled with learning a new language in a classroom or at home, try listening to audio instruction while on the road. Because of the extra blood flow triggered by exercise, researchers have found that learning ability and memory retention improves. You could be fluent in no time.

Spread happiness.

A friend of ours recently did an experiment. He started saying "hello" or waving to everyone he passed on his walks. And an interesting thing happened: Before long, people were greeting him first, and drivers even started giving him a wider berth. Try it.

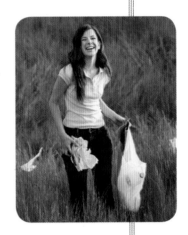

Beautify the neighborhood.

Instead of passing by the same trash on every walk, put on a pair of gloves and stuff the litter into a bag. The extra bending will provide an even better workout (or you can build a trash picker by attaching a nail to the end of a broomstick).

Become a "found artist."

The opportunity for art is everywhere; you just have to become aware. Strap on a small fanny pack and pick up interesting things you find along the way. Bits of colored glass, ticket stubs, Cracker Jack prizes, old coins, discarded shopping lists—all the interesting stuff that washes ashore daily on the tide of life. Once you have a sackful, try making a mosaic or—something else.

Become an intellectual.

TED is a nonprofit organization that challenges the world's most fascinating thinkers and doers to give the talk of their lives in 18 minutes. There are 700 of these speeches available for free download at ted.com/talks. The topics are diverse, provocative, and at the very least, ensure that you're never without something to say at cocktail parties.

Rehearse a speech.

Have an important presentation coming up? Rehearse it on the road. Talk out loud, use lots of hand gestures, and when you're finished, do a few forward bends to stretch those hamstring muscles (and, of course, practice your bow).

Solve all your problems.

Really. Here's how to do it: Before leaving on a walk, sit down and take five minutes to ponder the dilemma you're facing. Then head out the door and forget about it. Turn up the tunes and take your mind off it. Even though you won't be consciously cranking on it, your subconscious will be. And at some point during the walk, the solution will often pop into your head.

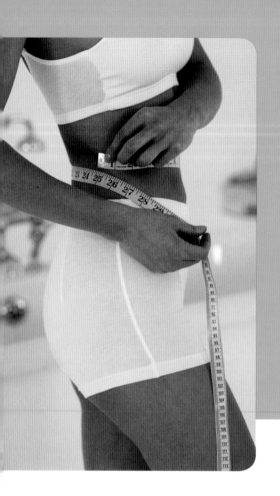

An *8-Week* Walking Plan

This 8-week walking plan focuses on two key goals: building endurance and burning fat—especially the dangerous fat lurking deep in your belly. On this plan, you'll build up to working out at 85 percent of your maximum heart rate for a few minutes at a time. Boosting your heart rate requires incorporating bursts of faster walking, hilly terrain, and aggressive arm pumping, which in turn will help you burn more fat. At the same time, you'll be introducing variety and increasing the amount of time and distance you're walking, ultimately building speed and endurance.

Week 1

DAY 1

5 minutes at 50% maximum heart rate (HR)
20 minutes at 60% maximum HR
10 minutes at 50% maximum HR **Total: 35 min**

DAY 2

5 minutes at 50% maximum HR
Repeat this sequence 5 times:
    1 minute at 60% maximum HR;
    1 minute at 70% maximum HR
10 minutes at 50% maximum HR **Total: 25 min**

DAY 3

5 minutes at 50% maximum HR
20 minutes at 60% maximum HR
10 minutes at 50% maximum HR **Total: 35 min**

DAY 4

5 minutes at 50% maximum HR
Repeat this sequence 5 times:
    1 minute at 60% maximum HR;
    1 minute at 70% maximum HR
10 minutes at 50% maximum HR **Total: 25 min**

DAY 5

5 minutes at 50% maximum HR
30 minutes at 60% maximum HR
10 minutes at 50% maximum HR **Total: 45 min**

MEDITATION IN MOTION

Walks are great times to take a mental retreat. Use the repetitive movement to keep your mind focused and away from your worries so you return from your walk refreshed. Concentrate on feeling each foot strike the ground and on breathing rhythmically in sync with your footfalls. As thoughts come to mind, allow them to pass on through.

Week 2

DAY 1

5 minutes at 50% maximum heart rate (HR)

10 minutes at 60% maximum HR

5 minutes at 70% maximum HR

10 minutes at 60% maximum HR

10 minutes at 50% maximum HR   **Total: 40 min**

DAY 2

5 minutes at 50% maximum HR

Repeat this sequence 5 times:

   1 minute at 60% maximum HR;

   1 minute at 70% maximum HR;

   1 minute at 80% maximum HR

10 minutes at 50% maximum HR   **Total: 30 min**

DAY 3

5 minutes at 50% maximum HR

10 minutes at 60% maximum HR

5 minutes at 70% maximum HR

10 minutes at 60% maximum HR

10 minutes at 50% maximum HR   **Total: 40 min**

DAY 4

5 minutes at 50% maximum HR

Repeat this sequence 5 times:

   1 minute at 60% maximum HR;

   1 minute at 70% maximum HR;

   1 minute at 80% maximum HR

10 minutes at 50% maximum HR   **Total: 30 min**

DAY 5

5 minutes at 50% maximum HR

35 minutes at 60% maximum HR

10 minutes at 50% maximum HR   **Total: 50 min**

Week 3

DAY 1

5 minutes at 50% maximum heart rate (HR)
5 minutes at 60% maximum HR
10 minutes at 70% maximum HR
5 minutes at 60% maximum HR
10 minutes at 50% maximum HR **Total: 35 min**

DAY 2

5 minutes at 50% maximum HR
Repeat this sequence 5 times:
   1 minute at 60% maximum HR;
   2 minutes at 80% maximum HR
10 minutes at 50% maximum HR **Total: 30 min**

DAY 3

5 minutes at 50% maximum HR
5 min at 60% maximum HR
10 minutes at 70% maximum HR
5 minutes at 60% maximum HR
10 minutes at 50% maximum HR **Total: 35 min**

DAY 4

5 minutes at 50% maximum HR
Repeat this sequence 5 times:
   1 minute at 60% maximum HR;
   2 minutes at 80% maximum HR
10 minutes at 50% maximum HR **Total: 30 min**

DAY 5

5 minutes at 50% maximum HR
40 minutes at 60% maximum HR
10 minutes at 50% maximum HR **Total: 55 min**

CALCULATE YOUR CALORIE BURN

There are cool gadgets ranging from pedometers, watch-style monitors, and smartphone apps that can help you estimate the calories you've burned.

But if you're not a gadget person, here's a rough guide: If you weigh 150 pounds and it takes you 30 minutes to walk a mile, you'll burn 95 calories in 30 minutes; if it takes you 20 minutes, you'll burn 130 calories in 30 minutes; if it takes you 15 minutes, you'll burn 187 calories in 30 minutes. If you weigh less, you'll burn less. If you weigh more, you'll burn more. Don't forget that by building more muscle, you're also boosting your metabolism for a more lasting payoff.

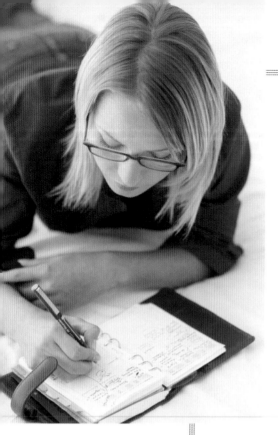

MAKE TIME TO WALK

Every day, you balance work, family, home, and a seemingly endless stream of errands and tasks. But why is it that devoting time to your own good health often doesn't make it on your to-do list? We've already established that walking is an easy, cheap (free!), year-round way to become the fit and healthy person you want to be. So get smart and plan for the time you need to get your life on a healthy track. Here's how:

Get out your planner and get creative.

Oftentimes, what seems a lack of time is actually lack of prioritizing. Start by sitting down with your planner. If you don't use one, get out a notepad and sketch out what every day during the week looks like, including what time you get up, what time you go to sleep, and everything in between. As best you can, account for everything from watching the nightly news to driving the carpool.

Then dust off the same problem-solving skills you use at work or with the kids and look for places where you might trade one activity for another. Can you watch 30 minutes of TV each night instead of 60 and use a slice of that time to exercise or put together a salad for tomorrow's lunch—or walk on the treadmill while you watch? Can you bring lunch to work three days a week rather than two, giving you time to sneak in one more walk at work? Can your kids take the bus to school a couple of days a week or carpool to get to sports games, leaving you free to do chores so you can get to bed on time? Where there's a will, there's a way.

Build in time for sleep.

If your solution to "getting it all done" is to stay up later—or you're so wiped out while watching TV at night that you're too tired to get up and turn the thing off—it's time to enforce a strict bedtime. Lack of sleep ratchets up stress hormones, which make life seem that much more out of control. It also contributes more than you might think to a wide waistline. A Canadian study of 740 adults found that people who reported getting five to six hours of sleep a night were 38 percent more likely to be overweight than those getting seven to eight hours.

If you're having trouble holding yourself to a bedtime, buy timers for the TV and all the lights in your living room. Set them to turn off at 10:30 P.M. or earlier. Or set a reminder on your computer to ring at 10:15 P.M.—an alert that time is almost up. Bonus: Once your body gets used to going to bed at the same time every night (even on weekends!), you'll fall asleep faster.

Practice the art of delegation.

Enlist your spouse and kids to help you make the best use of your time. If handing over certain responsibilities doesn't work at first, stick with it. "Initially it can take more time to delegate than to do the task yourself," admits Peggy Duncan, an organizational consultant based in Atlanta and author of *The Time Management Memory Jogger*. "But if you invest a little time to teach others how to complete tasks, and then hold them accountable, the jobs will get done." You might be frustrated if your husband doesn't fold the laundry exactly the way you do, or if your children put the forks on the right of the plate when they set the table, but remember: The trade-off is a valuable 10 or 20 minutes of time you can devote to yourself. What's more, "Including children in the responsibility of running the household can make them feel more grown-up," says Sternberg.

How do you get your gang on board? Write up a list of the household chores for which each person is responsible, and put it on the fridge. Be sure to include your own tasks — all the ones you already do. Since your list will probably be the longest, no one else will have a leg to stand on if they decide to complain about being asked to pitch in.

Start every day off right.

Even though morning can be the most hectic part of your day, and you doubt you can find five minutes for breakfast, consider this double whammy: Skipping breakfast increases your risk for obesity and makes you less able to resist fatty and high-calorie foods later in the day. Make a vow to eat breakfast every day. It's a proven way to maintain a healthy body weight. A bowl of oatmeal or yogurt, topped with strawberries or blueberries and a sprinkling of ground flaxseed, starts you out with the complex carbohydrates, fiber, and protein you need to get you up and running.

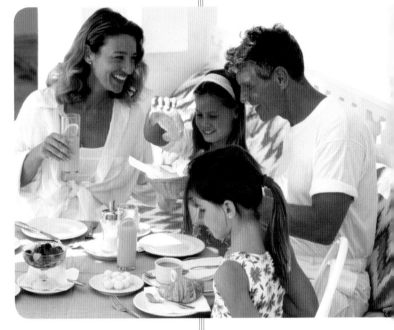

If you're trying to lose weight, putting some lean protein on your plate (or in a glass) is your best bet, according to results from a 2007 study. Researchers at the Pennington Biomedical Research Center compared weight loss in women who ate either two eggs or a plain bagel. The women who ate two eggs for breakfast five times a week for eight weeks as part of a low-fat, reduced-calorie diet lost 65 percent more weight than the women who ate bagels—even though they consumed the same number of calories. They also reported higher energy levels.

Plan a week's worth of dinners at a time.

All of a sudden it's four o'clock and you have no idea what's for dinner. Sound familiar? You're in good company: Research has shown that the majority of people don't know what they're having either. And lack of planning is probably what leads you to the drive-through or has you dialing for takeout. Both options can sabotage your health (and budget). A better idea is to keep a few go-to dinner recipes—ideally ones that your spouse or teenager can prepare—in a kitchen folder, and keep the key ingredients for them on hand in the pantry and freezer. Think "one-pot" meals like chicken stir-fry, pork chops with cabbage, or pasta with white beans and spinach.

Another time saver: Sit down on Saturday or Sunday and plan out your dinners for the week. Make a list of all the ingredients you'll need for each one, and—*voilà*—that's your shopping list. "If you have a list, you won't wander the aisles aimlessly," says Duncan. You can also take meal planning to a new level and devote two hours on a weekend afternoon to preparing several meals you'll eat later in the week. "You'll be shocked at how much time you'll free up and how much less stress you'll feel at dinnertime come midweek," says Duncan, who adopted the "cook ahead" tip from her mother.

Week 4

DAY 1

5 minutes at 50% maximum heart rate (HR)

5 minutes at 60% maximum HR

15 minutes at 70% maximum HR

5 minutes at 60% maximum HR

10 minutes at 50% maximum HR **Total: 40 min**

DAY 2

5 minutes at 50% maximum HR

Repeat this sequence 7 times:

    1 minute at 60% maximum HR;

    2 minutes at 80% maximum HR

9 minutes at 50% maximum HR **Total: 35 min**

DAY 3

5 minutes at 50% maximum HR

5 minutes at 60% maximum HR

15 minutes at 70% maximum HR

5 minutes at 60% maximum HR

10 minutes at 50% maximum HR **Total: 40 min**

DAY 4

5 minutes at 50% maximum HR

Repeat this sequence 7 times:

    1 minute at 60% maximum HR;

    2 minutes at 80% maximum HR

9 minutes at 50% maximum HR **Total: 35 min**

DAY 5

5 minutes at 50% maximum HR

45 minutes at 60% maximum HR

10 minutes at 50% maximum HR **Total: 60 min**

Week 5

DAY 1

5 minutes at 50% maximum heart rate (HR)

5 minutes at 60% maximum HR

20 minutes at 70% maximum HR

5 minutes at 60% maximum HR

5 minutes at 50% maximum HR   **Total: 40 min**

DAY 2

5 minutes at 50% maximum HR

Repeat this sequence 6 times:
    1 minute at 60% maximum HR;
    2 minutes at 80% maximum HR;
    1 minute at 85% maximum HR

11 minutes at 50% maximum HR   **Total: 40 min**

DAY 3

5 minutes at 50% maximum HR

5 minutes at 60% maximum HR

20 minutes at 70% maximum HR

5 minutes at 60% maximum HR

5 minutes at 50% maximum HR   **Total: 40 min**

DAY 4

5 minutes at 50% maximum HR

Repeat this sequence 6 times:
    1 minute at 60% maximum HR;
    2 minutes at 80% maximum HR;
    1 minute at 85% maximum HR

11 min at 50% maximum HR   **Total: 40 min**

DAY 5

5 minutes at 50% maximum HR

40 minutes at 65% maximum HR

10 minutes at 50% maximum HR   **Total: 55 min**

FASTER WALKING 101

Want to pick up the pace? Think short strides. One of the most common mistakes people make is lengthening their strides to walk faster. When you do, your front foot acts like a brake, jarring your joints and slowing you down. Instead, take short, quick heel-to-toe strides.

Week 6

DAY 1

5 minutes at 50% maximum heart rate (HR)
5 minutes at 60% maximum HR
25 minutes at 70% maximum HR
5 minutes at 60% maximum HR
5 minutes at 50% maximum HR   **Total: 45 min**

DAY 2

5 minutes at 50% maximum HR
Repeat this sequence 7 times:
    1 minute at 65% maximum HR;
    2 minutes at 80% maximum HR
9 minutes at 50% maximum HR   **Total: 35 min**

DAY 3

5 minutes at 50% maximum HR
5 minutes at 60% maximum HR
25 minutes at 70% maximum HR
10 minutes at 50% maximum HR   **Total: 45 min**

DAY 4

5 minutes at 50% maximum HR
Repeat this sequence 7 times:
    1 minute at 65% maximum HR;
    2 minutes at 80% maximum HR
9 minutes at 50% maximum HR   **Total: 35 min**

DAY 5

5 minutes at 50% maximum HR
45 minutes at 65% maximum HR
10 minutes at 50% maximum HR   **Total: 60 min**

Week 7

DAY 1

5 minutes at 50% maximum heart rate (HR)
5 minutes at 60% maximum HR
30 minutes at 70% maximum HR
5 minutes at 60% maximum HR
5 minutes at 50% maximum HR   **Total: 50 min**

DAY 2

5 minutes at 50% maximum HR
Repeat this sequence 6 times:
    1 minute at 65% maximum HR;
    2 minutes at 80% maximum HR;
    1 minute at 85% maximum HR
11 minutes at 50% maximum HR   **Total: 40 min**

DAY 3

5 minutes at 50% maximum HR
5 minutes at 60% maximum HR
30 minutes at 70% maximum HR
5 minutes at 60% maximum HR
5 minutes at 50% maximum HR   **Total: 50 min**

DAY 4

5 minutes at 50% maximum HR
Repeat this sequence 6 times:
    1 minute at 65% maximum HR;
    2 minute at 80% maximum HR;
    1 min at 85% maximum HR
11 minutes at 50% maximum HR   **Total: 40 min**

DAY 5

5 minutes at 50% maximum HR
50 minutes at 65% maximum HR
10 minutes at 50% maximum HR   **Total: 65 min**

GREAT GADGETS

Pedometer

What can you buy for as little as six bucks that could potentially transform your weight loss from so-so to go-go? Most pedometers are smaller than a pack of gum and clip easily to a waistband. (You can also buy a watch that doubles as a pedometer.) Put one on in the morning, and almost magically you'll find yourself moving more

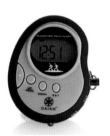

during the day. In fact, one study showed that people who wore a pedometer increased their daily steps by a whopping 27 percent.

It's like the food-diary phenomenon: Just as the simple act of writing down what foods you eat makes you choose foods more carefully, so does the simple fact of knowing how many steps you're taking in a day make you try to take more, whether it's by parking farther from your destination or adding an extra block to your daily walk.

To get the most from your pedometer, set a goal. To do this, determine the average number of daily steps you take now, then multiply this number by 1.2 to determine your goal. Once you've set your goal, track your progress. Study subjects who did this, either by writing down the number of steps they took each day or uploading that number onto an electronic exercise diary, moved more than people who didn't keep track. Compare your numbers against your weekly goal and make daily adjustments to stay on track. To set your next week's goal, multiply your new average number of steps by 1.2.

MP3 Player

Want to walk longer or harder without even noticing? Bring your MP3 player along. Studies show that listening to music helps you exercise harder with less perceived effort by distracting you from your feelings of exertion.

There's no magic formula for constructing your optimal playlist; just select songs well matched to your pace. Many fitness enthusiasts post free workout-specific podcasts on iTunes (or you can download some at www.fitpod.com), and many iTunes songs list beats per minute so you

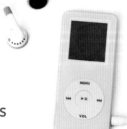

can select the right tempo for your workout.

Walking Poles

It sounds like one of those too-good-to-be-true infomercials: Burn more calories without even trying! Except for this time, the claim is true. The products are walking poles, not far off from the ones used in cross-country skiing. If you're prone to knee problems, walking poles can help you take on hills. And if you really get those poles swinging as you walk, you can up your caloric expenditure by as much as 40 percent. Best of all, in one study people who used the poles burned more calories yet didn't feel like they were working any harder than they had without the poles.

Walking poles began as a way for hikers to get some extra traction on the uphills and take some strain off their joints on steep descents. But a new generation of so-called Nordic

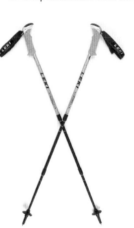

walking poles are designed for use on any terrain, even sidewalks. Special pole tips offer traction on pavement or dirt. Nordic poles are lighter than traditional hiking poles, and they come with grips designed to help you activate more upper-body muscles. Poles should hit at about elbow height, and many models are adjustable. Another bonus: Because walking with poles gets your upper body and torso in on the act, you tone your arms, shoulders, and core muscles without lifting a single dumbbell.

Nordic walking technique is simple: Keep your hip bones facing forward and swing your arms in synch with your legs—as you move your left leg, reach forward with your right arm and plant your pole near your foot. (See also "Great Gear to Step Out In," page 210.)

Week 8

DAY 1

5 minutes at 50% maximum heart rate (HR)

5 minutes at 60% maximum HR

15 minutes at 70% maximum HR

5 minutes at 80% maximum HR

15 minutes at 70% maximum HR

5 minutes at 60% maximum HR

5 minutes at 50% maximum HR   **Total: 55 min**

DAY 2

5 minutes at 50% maximum HR

Repeat this sequence 7 times:

    1 minute at 65% maximum HR;

    3 minutes at 80% maximum HR

12 minutes at 50% maximum HR   **Total: 45 min**

DAY 3

5 minutes at 50% maximum HR

5 minutes at 60% maximum HR

15 minutes at 70% maximum HR

5 minutes at 80% maximum HR

15 minutes at 70% maximum HR

5 minutes at 60% maximum HR

5 minutes at 50% maximum HR   **Total: 55 min**

DAY 4

5 minutes at 50% maximum HR

Repeat this sequence 7 times:

    1 minute at 65% maximum HR;

    3 minutes at 80% maximum HR

12 minutes at 50% maximum HR   **Total: 45 min**

DAY 5

5 minutes at 50% maximum HR

55 minutes at 65% maximum HR

10 minutes at 50% maximum HR   **Total: 70 min**

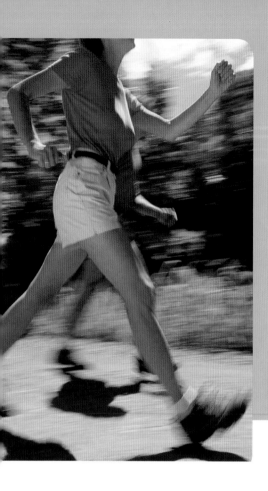

Step It Up

It won't take long to fall in love with walking—

the energy it gives you, the way it buoys your mood, the feeling you get from becoming fitter with every step. But if you're walking to lose weight, chances are you'd like to see those pounds come off faster.

Most people quickly drop a pound or three when they start a new walking program, but after a few months weight loss tends to slow down, and it's not unusual to hit a sticking point. Often this weight-loss plateau is a symptom of success: As you get fit, your body becomes more efficient at walking, allowing you to walk farther with less effort—and fewer calories burned. To keep the weight loss coming, you'll need to step up your routine.

Cutting calories from your diet and hitting the weight room to build metabolism-boosting muscle are two surefire ways to speed your progress. But nothing will help you crank your walks up a notch more than interval training—incorporating short bursts of harder efforts into your regular workout. For years elite runners and race walkers have used this secret strategy to boost performance, and now you can use it to turbocharge your weight loss.

The concept is simple: The harder you walk, the more calories you burn. Now, you certainly don't want to go all-out on your entire walk or you'll be exhausted (and maybe even injured) in no time. But you can still reap the weight-loss benefits of high-intensity workouts by throwing in brief bouts of faster walking along the way. You'll not only speed your weight loss, but also give your fitness gains a giant boost—without adding a single extra minute to your time on the pavement.

Scientists have discovered that to shed the most fat, you should walk at an intensity of at least 3 METs, a scientific way of saying that you're moving quickly enough to meaningfully raise your heart rate, increase your body's need for oxygen, and combust calories. 1 MET, or Metabolic Equivalent of Task, equals burning 1 calorie per kilogram of body weight per hour (if you weigh 180 pounds, that's 81 kilograms, or 81 calories per hour).

Just how fast do you need to walk to reach 3 METS? Researchers at San Diego State University set out to answer that. They asked 97 men and women to walk on treadmills as they measured their METs and counted their steps. In the end, they found that the magic number is 100 steps per minute (spm). That's the minimum you need for calorie-burning aerobic benefit. To lose fat faster, you need to step quicker.

"Taking quicker steps is the opposite of what many people do when they're trying to get more from their walking workouts," says Leigh Crews, national spokesperson for the American Council on Exercise and general manager of Club Fitness in Rome, Georgia, who helped develop the walking programs presented here. Many people try for longer strides, which actually slows them down and uses fewer muscles.

If you really want to see your walking program pay off, you'll need to eat smart, too. So while the occasional "reward treat" is fine, limit yourself to a healthy diet filled with fresh fruits, vegetables, lean proteins, healthful fats (think fish and olive oil), and whole grains. Now let's get down to some walking.

Walk It Off PLAYLIST

Country

"Need You Now,"
Lady Antebellum

"Mine,"
Taylor Swift

"Crazy,"
Patsy Cline

"Cowboy Casanova,"
Carrie Underwood

"Hillbilly Bone,"
Blake Shelton with
Trace Adkins

"Ring of Fire,"
Johnny Cash

"The Dance,"
Garth Brooks

"Wide Open Spaces,"
The Dixie Chicks

"Always On My Mind,"
Willie Nelson

"Kiss a Girl,"
Keith Urban

Quick-Step Weight Loss

To get the most benefit from your roadwork, use the 100 steps-per-minute mark as a baseline then add bursts of faster stepping to rev your results. Research shows that interval training yields significantly faster weight loss than one-speed workouts. Most remarkably, a study from the University of South Wales found that women who exercised 3 days per week for 20 minutes, alternating fast- and moderate-paced intervals, lost 5 times more weight (up to 18 pounds in 15 weeks without changing their diet) than those who exercised at a steady, brisk speed for twice that amount of time. As if that isn't exciting enough, the interval exercisers sliced most of their fat from stubborn spots such as the legs and belly.

To get yourself moving more quickly, steal some tips from racewalkers. Did you ever notice how a racewalker's body angles are kind of sharp? The elbows are bent at

90 degrees, as is the knee on the front leg until it makes contact with the ground. This is aerodynamics helping to propel the racewalker forward. As she walks, the racewalker's bent elbows shorten the pendulum action of the swinging arms, enabling the arms to swing more quickly and drive the body forward. At the same time, she's pushing purposefully off the rear toes, which helps to drive the knee forward.

These two simple actions—bending the elbows and explosively pushing off with the back foot—combine to push your body forward faster. Before you begin to integrate interval programs into your walks, practice this technique for short distances—no more than 30 seconds or so, with a minimum of two minutes of regular walking in between—during your regular walks.

Keep your neck, shoulders, and hands relaxed, not tense or clenched. Swing your arms loosely but vigorously, and keep your hands and elbows close to your body. Lead with your heel, then roll right through to push off with your toes. Notice the difference between your ordinary pace and what happens when you make like a racewalker. It may feel awkward at first, but practice it until the movement feels smooth and natural. And now you're ready to get with the interval workout plan.

The Plan

The three interval workouts are based on these three paces:

- **Base Pace:** 100–115 spm (3–3.3 m.p.h.)
- **Burn Pace:** 115–130 spm (3.3–3.8 m.p.h.)
- **Power Pace:** 130–145 spm (3.8–4.5 m.p.h.)

Do the interval workouts three days per week (a different workout each day), preferably on non-consecutive days so your body can rest and recover in between. On alternate days, walk at Base to Burn Pace for 30 to 60 minutes. Take one day off per week.

If you're walking on a treadmill, feel free to use m.p.h. instead of steps per minute (s.p.m.).

WHAT'S YOUR S.P.M.?

Calculating your steps-per-minute (s.p.m.) is as easy as it sounds—just count. For the best results, warm up for a few minutes. Then, using the second hand on your watch, count how many steps you take in one minute. (You can also count your steps for 20 seconds and multiply by 3.) Whatever method you choose, repeat it three times and take the average. If your number is below 100, pick up the pace and repeat the test until you're in the 100–115 s.p.m. range. Every time you begin walking, count your steps again until that pace becomes second nature. Repeat this process with faster step counts in order to feel what it's like to walk 115–130 s.p.m. and 130–145 s.p.m.

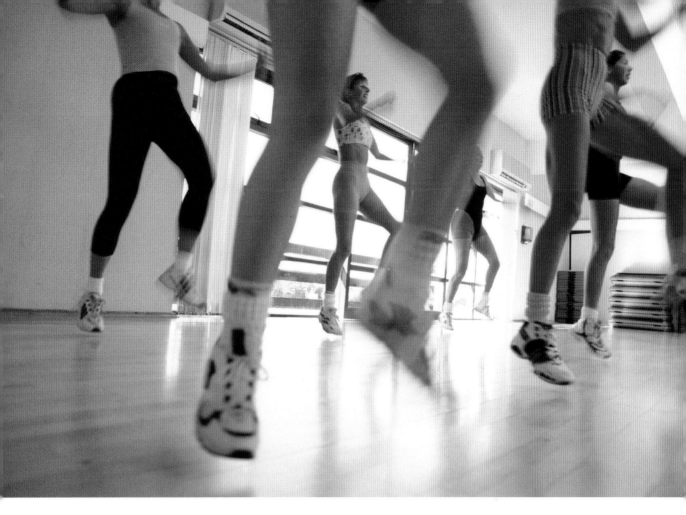

INTERVAL WORKOUT #1

Double Downs

These high-energy intervals are hard (but not exhausting), so you fry lots of fat, strengthen your heart, and boost overall fitness while still reserving energy for all your other daily duties. You'll do 4 minutes at Burn Pace (aiming for the high end of the range), followed by 2 minutes at Base Pace. After 5 weeks, increase the amount of time at Burn Pace to 6 minutes and recover for 3 minutes at Base Pace. Here is a sample 40-minute workout:

Start	Warm up, working to Base Pace
4:00	Burn Pace
8:00	Base Pace
10:00	Repeat minutes 4 through 10 four more times
34:00	Cool down, from the top to the low range of Base Pace
40:00	Finish

MOVE TO THE MUSIC

It's no coincidence that aerobic instructors have been carefully selecting dance mixes since, well, there have been aerobic instructors. A music's tempo, or beats per minute (bpm), can keep you moving at your desired pace without even thinking about it. Most commercial dance music, from classic Madonna to Rihanna, has a tempo ranging from 120 to 140 bpm, which is perfect for quick-step, weight-loss intervals.

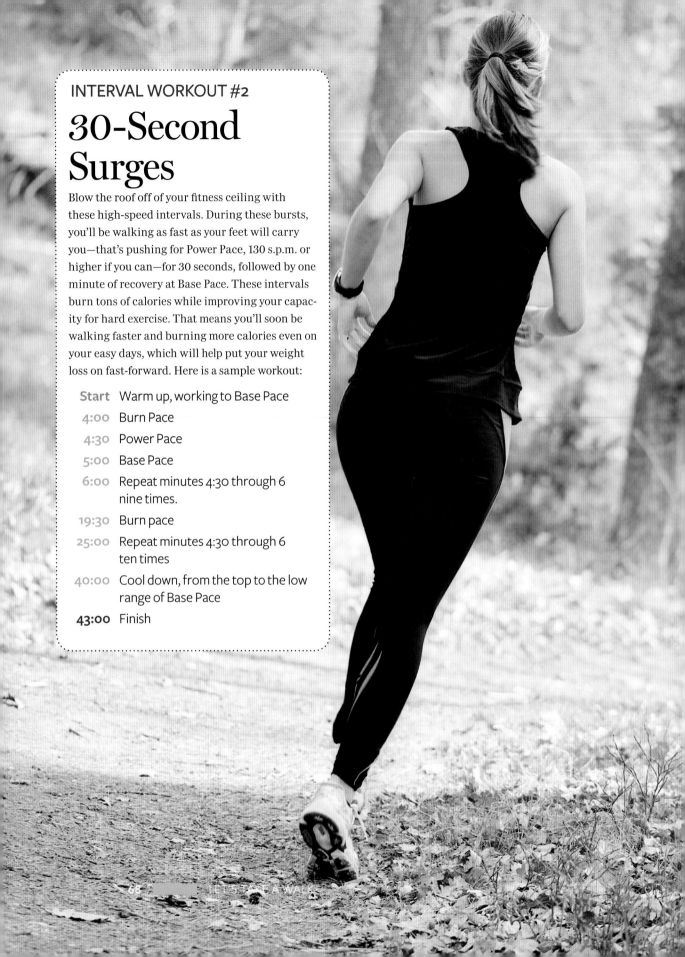

INTERVAL WORKOUT #2

30-Second Surges

Blow the roof off of your fitness ceiling with these high-speed intervals. During these bursts, you'll be walking as fast as your feet will carry you—that's pushing for Power Pace, 130 s.p.m. or higher if you can—for 30 seconds, followed by one minute of recovery at Base Pace. These intervals burn tons of calories while improving your capacity for hard exercise. That means you'll soon be walking faster and burning more calories even on your easy days, which will help put your weight loss on fast-forward. Here is a sample workout:

Start	Warm up, working to Base Pace
4:00	Burn Pace
4:30	Power Pace
5:00	Base Pace
6:00	Repeat minutes 4:30 through 6 nine times.
19:30	Burn pace
25:00	Repeat minutes 4:30 through 6 ten times
40:00	Cool down, from the top to the low range of Base Pace
43:00	Finish

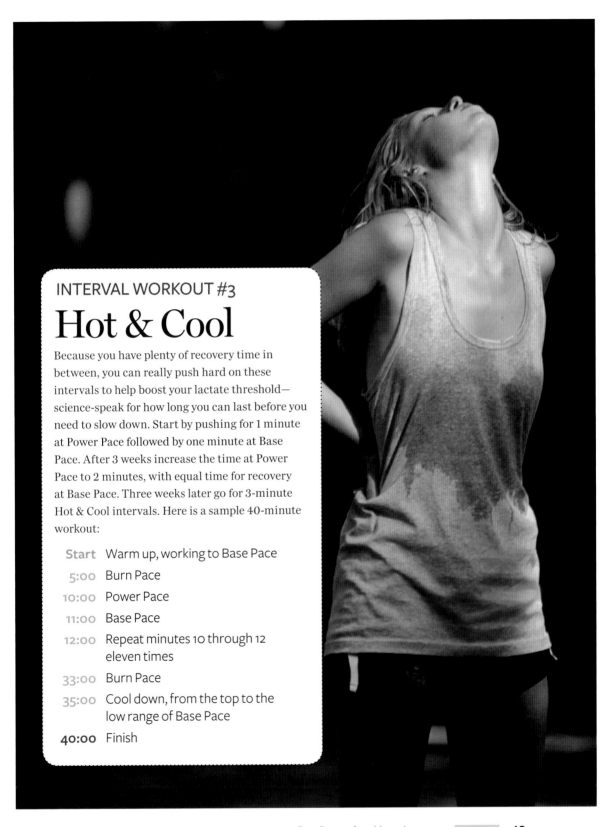

INTERVAL WORKOUT #3

Hot & Cool

Because you have plenty of recovery time in between, you can really push hard on these intervals to help boost your lactate threshold—science-speak for how long you can last before you need to slow down. Start by pushing for 1 minute at Power Pace followed by one minute at Base Pace. After 3 weeks increase the time at Power Pace to 2 minutes, with equal time for recovery at Base Pace. Three weeks later go for 3-minute Hot & Cool intervals. Here is a sample 40-minute workout:

Start	Warm up, working to Base Pace
5:00	Burn Pace
10:00	Power Pace
11:00	Base Pace
12:00	Repeat minutes 10 through 12 eleven times
33:00	Burn Pace
35:00	Cool down, from the top to the low range of Base Pace
40:00	Finish

TONE ON THE GO

Intervals will help you burn fat and build some muscle, but to really firm as you burn, it helps to strength-train, which adds even more metabolism-revving muscle. Here are five exercises you can do during (if it's not an interval day) your walks.

Park Presses

TONES YOUR CHEST, TRICEPS, SHOULDERS, AND CORE

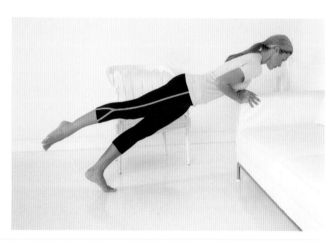

Stand facing the back of a park bench or low wall (or if indoors, the arm or back of a couch). Place both hands on the bench shoulder-width apart and walk your feet back until you're balancing on the balls of your feet and your body forms a straight line from head to heels.

Lift your right foot so your toes are a few inches off the ground. From that position, slowly bend your elbows and lower your chest toward bench until your elbows are in line with your shoulders.

Pause a second and then slowly push back up. Repeat 10–15 times. Next set, lift the opposite foot.

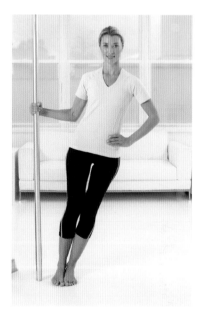

Pole Side Pulls

TONES YOUR ARMS AND CORE

Stand to the immediate right of a flagpole or skinny tree (or if indoors, use a pole, stairway spindle, or the handle of a securely closed door). Grasp it with your right hand, and lean toward the left until your right arm is nearly extended.

Slowly bend your right elbow and pull your body back until you're almost standing vertically and then slowly drop back again.

Repeat 20 times then switch sides.

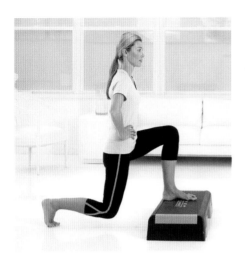

Curb Lunge

TONES YOUR GLUTES, THIGHS, AND HIPS

Stand about 3 feet away from and facing a curb (or if indoors, 3 feet in front of a secure step). Place your hands on your hips. Step forward with your left foot and place it on the curb so your knee is directly over your ankle.

Keeping your body upright, bend both knees and drop toward the ground until your front thigh is parallel to the ground. Step back to start and repeat to the opposite side. That's one rep. Do 10–15 reps.

To exercise your oblique muscles at the same time, you can rotate your torso in the direction of your front foot as you lower.

Bench Dip

TONES YOUR ARMS, SHOULDERS, AND UPPER BACK

Sit on the edge of a bench (or if indoors, a stable chair) with your hands grasping the seat on either side of your hips. Bend your legs 90 degrees with your feet flat on the floor. Slide your behind off the seat and walk your feet forward slightly, maintaining the 90-degree angle with your legs.

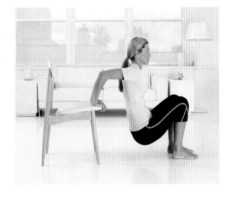

Keeping shoulders down, bend your elbows straight back, lowering your hips toward the ground until your upper arms are nearly parallel to the ground.

Press back to the starting position. Try 10–15 of these.

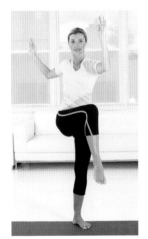

Standing Crisscross

TONES YOUR ABS AND OBLIQUES

Stand with your feet a few inches apart. Bend your arms and hold them out to the sides so they form right angles with hands pointing toward the sky, palms facing forward.

Contract your abs and pull your right knee and left elbow toward one another.

Pause and return to start position. Do 10–15, then switch sides.

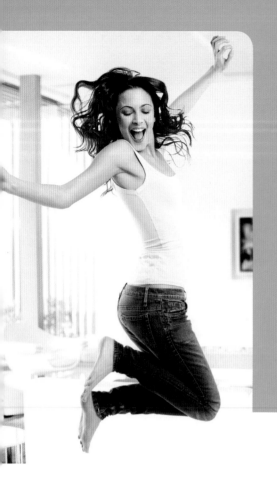

Add Energy to Your Stride

Losing weight is only partly about exercise and eating right. It's also about establishing habits that optimize your energy, alertness, and mindfulness throughout the day.

Simple Habits to Keep You Going

Carrying extra pounds is tiring, and even though walking 30 minutes a day gives you an energy boost that lasts for hours, you may need even more energy to get through your day. Try a handful of these quick-and-easy tips designed to boost your get-up-and-go.

Sip "short" cups of coffee throughout the day. Do you down a triple shot of espresso just to bring your eyelids to half-mast in the morning? You may be inadvertently driving yourself deeper into a low-energy rut. Research from Harvard Medical School finds that frequent low doses of caffeine (the amount in a quarter cup of coffee) are more effective than a few larger doses in keeping people alert.

Lighten your glycemic load. Foods with a low glycemic load, like beans, bran cereal, barley, nuts, and yogurt, have less impact on your blood sugar than foods that are high glycemic: like white rice, spaghetti, potatoes, cornflakes, baked goods, and sugary juices and drinks. Eating more low-glycemic foods will help keep your blood sugar steady and avoid the lightheadedness and "shakes" associated with blood sugar drops, which usually follow spikes.

Slip in some strides. Sneak in a brisk 10-minute walk when you're feeling sluggish. Often, people with fatigue have a decreased supply of adenosine diphosphate (ADP), an intracellular "messenger" involved in energy metabolism. Translation: There's not enough "spark" in the engine. So jump-start it with a brief jaunt.

Walk gratefully. As you stride, focus on what you feel most thankful for. "This simple technique combines the power of gratefulness with the positive effects of walking and exercise, flooding your brain with happy neurotransmitters and endorphins," says Jon Gordon, energy coach and author of *Become an Energy Addict*. "It's a simple yet powerful exercise that energizes the mind and body."

Chug two glasses of icy water. Fatigue is often one of the first symptoms of dehydration, and if all you've sipped all day is coffee and soft drinks, it's quite likely you're dehydrated. Plus, the refreshing coldness will serve as a virtual slap in the face.

Try Siberian ginseng. This herbal remedy stimulates your nervous system and may help to protect your body from the ravages of stress. Look for a supplement containing at least 4 percent ginsenosides, and take two 100-mg capsules daily. Caveat: Ginseng is off-limits if you have high blood pressure.

GINSENG CAN STIMULATE YOUR NERVOUS SYSTEM AND MAY HELP PROTECT YOUR BODY FROM STRESS.

Have your thyroid checked. If it's not producing enough thyroid hormone, it could be making you feel tired and run down. A simple blood test will tell. Other symptoms of low thyroid are dry skin, weight gain, constipation, and feeling cold.

Turn in 15 minutes early. Every week go to bed an additional 15 minutes earlier until you find the right amount of sleep for your body. You'll know you've had enough when you wake up feeling refreshed.

Wake up on time. Rules apply to mornings as well. Wake up at the same time every day, even on weekends, no matter how little sleep you get the night before. By forcing your body to adhere to the pattern, you'll fall asleep faster when your head hits the pillow. Give it a few weeks to work.

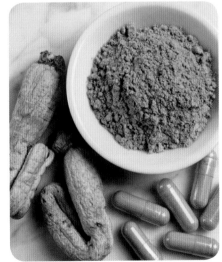

Fill up on phosphorus. Phosphorus is an essential mineral the body needs to metabolize carbohydrates, fat, and protein so they can be used as energy. Add a little here and a little there to your diet from this list of the top 10 sources of phosphorus to boost your energy: bran (rice and oat); pumpkin, squash, and sunflower seeds; toasted wheat germ; Parmesan cheese; sesame seeds; nuts (Brazil and pine); roasted soybeans (edamame); flaxseed; and bacon.

Eat every four hours. It's much better to continually refuel your body before it hits empty than to wait until you're in the danger zone and then overdo it. So every four hours (except, of course, when you're sleeping) have a mini meal or snack. This could be a bowl of whole-grain cereal—or a handful of roasted peanuts with a hard-boiled egg or slice of lean luncheon meat, and a sliced apple.

Get screened for depression. Feeling fatigued and tired regardless of how much you're sleeping is a primary symptom of depression. Ask your doctor to administer a depression screening test, or simply answer the following two questions, which studies find are excellent indicators for predicting depression: 1) Over the past two weeks, have you felt down, depressed, or hopeless? And 2) Over the past two weeks, have you felt little interest or pleasure in doing things? If you answered yes to these questions, see your doctor for a more complete examination.

Replace your pillow. More restful, reinvigorating sleep may be within your reach quite literally—if you upgrade your pillow. Wake up in the morning with a sore neck? Opt for a soft, thinner pillow or a special "neck pillow." In one Swedish study a neck pillow enhanced sleep. These pillows come in different shapes—some are rolls, others are rectangular with a depression in the middle.

Supplement with roseroot. *Rhodiola rosea,* also called roseroot, can help you better manage stress and zap fatigue. Doses of 200 to 600 mg a day are typical, but check with your doc first about possible interactions with other medications.

Breathe in energy. Sit in a chair with a straight back, place your hands over your stomach, and breathe into your belly so that your hands rise and fall with your breath. Imagine you're inhaling a white light that fills your body with vital energy. Do this for five full breaths. Then, as you inhale, tighten the muscles that connect your shoulders and neck, pulling your shoulders up toward your ears. "When your shoulders are snug around your ears, hold your breath for

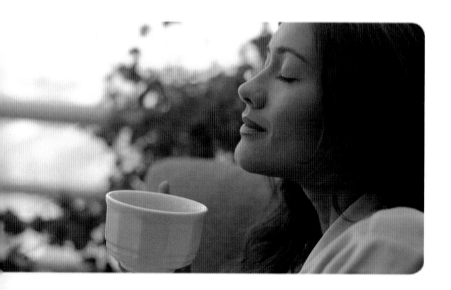

just a second," says Karl D. La Rowe, a licensed clinical social worker in Oregon. "Then exhale as you release the tension and your breath in one big whoosh— as though you're releasing the weight of the world from your shoulders. Repeat until you feel refreshed and revitalized."

Take a multi. Research at the University of California at Berkeley found that the amino acid L-carnitine and the antioxidant alpha-lipoic acid can boost both memory and energy, possibly by improving the way body cells produce energy. Bruce Ames, PhD, one

EMERGENCY ENERGY

Really in need of some extra energy fast? Resort to this trick: Drink a cup of coffee, then lie down for a 30-minute nap (set your alarm). By the time you wake up, you'll be energized from the nap—and the caffeine will start kicking in. Use this strategy for emergencies only. In general, experts say that if fatigue is a problem for you, you're better off skipping caffeine altogether.

of the study authors, says you can consume the right amount of both nutrients by taking a daily multivitamin and eating a diet rich in colorful fruits and veggies.

Get inclined. Lie on your back and use pillows to prop up your feet so they're higher than your head, or better yet, lie on an adjustable exercise bench or other surface that slants. In India yogis do this to encourage blood flow to the brain, which is thought to fight fatigue and boost alertness.

Head for the Hills

It's basic physics: Hefting your body uphill takes more energy than walking on flat ground. In fact, depending on the slope, walking uphill burns two to four times the calories as walking on a walking on a flat surface. It also tones your butt, calves, and core muscles. What you might not know about walking uphill is how it helps to put a spring in all of the rest of your steps every day by strengthening (and toning) your butt, calves, and core muscles. That's right—incorporating hills into your walking can make all of your walking more energetic and help you burn more calories and fat, with all of those great muscles you're building.

An ideal walking hill is steep enough to boost your effort level without leaving you breathless and unable to keep going. If you live in hill country, you may have such terrain in your neighborhood. If not, check out nearby state parks or wildlife areas. In a pinch you can usually find a set of shallow stairs, like those leading to public buildings, somewhere along your walk; take advantage and do a few vertical laps.

The slope of the hill will dictate how you integrate it into your workout. If possible, warm up on a flat stretch, then start your ascent. On long, gradual hills aim for a steady pace. On short, steep hills focus on pushing yourself up and over the top, where you can reward yourself by easing up to catch your breath.

What goes up must come down, and even walking downhill can increase your

The Power Surge. Not a sprint, but simply a surge in speed. Aim for one notch above your comfort zone—slow enough that you could talk if you had to, but hard enough to feel your breathing. To do this, start at your regular pace, then surge for 30 seconds. Add one or two of these surges during your walk. As you progress, add a third. If you don't want to look at your watch, count steps instead, substituting seconds for steps.

The Pyramid. A gradual increase in effort. You'll begin at an easy pace and finish at your top speed. Simply start at a leisurely rate. After 15 seconds increase your pace slightly.

Continue for 15 more seconds, then up your pace again and maintain it for 15 more seconds. Finish with 15 seconds of near-all-out effort. As you progress, aim to integrate several pyramids into your walk, with plenty of slower walking in between.

The Speed Blast. A quick burst of hard walking. You should be breathing too hard to carry on a conversation. Pick a landmark up ahead or give yourself 20 seconds on your watch and challenge yourself to push hard until time's up. If you often walk the same route, make of habit of speed blasting to familiar landmarks, such as stop signs or a favorite tree.

Walk It Off PLAYLIST

Hip-Hop

"Lose Yourself,"
Eminem

"Scenario,"
A Tribe Called Quest

"Find Your Love,"
Drake

"Protect Ya Neck,"
Wu Tang Clan

"Walk it Out,"
DJ UNK

"Stronger,"
Kanye West

"Slam,"
Onyx (Boom Box Flava)

"Check It Out,"
will.i.am with Nicki Minaj

"In Da Club,"
50 Cent

"Here I Come,"
The Roots

calorie burn. When you descend a steep incline, muscles in your legs and torso must work overtime to control your downward momentum and keep your body upright.

Whether you're walking uphill or down, technique matters. When going up, shorten your stride and lean ever so slightly into the hill, taking care to keep your shoulders and hips in alignment—avoid bending at the waist. Swinging your arms can help you propel yourself up the hill. When walking downhill, you can lengthen your stride a tad if the grade isn't too steep, but focus on keeping your knees and hips relaxed and avoid leaning too far forward or back.

No Hill? No Problem

Even flatlanders can hit the hills. Most gym treadmills (and even many mid-range home models) come with an adjustable incline. Most inclines start at 1 percent and go up to about 12 percent. Here's how to use inclines:

- Warm up for 5 to 10 minutes on a 0 or 1 percent grade.
- Gradually increase the incline. You can either work up to the maximum incline by walking 1 to 5 minutes at each incline setting, then moving up to the next level, or you can perform a hill interval workout by switching back and forth between walking 1 to 5 minutes at a steep incline (5 percent or more) and 1 to 5 minutes at a slighter incline (1 to 4 percent).
- To really make your calorie burn soar, walk at an incline of 5 to 7 percent. You'll feel the extra load in your hamstrings and quadriceps. When the grade reaches 7 percent or more, your effort will start to mimic hiking and your glutes and calves will get a killer workout.

Keep It Up

Sometimes you just need to use your head to keep your energy up, your motivation high, and your eating habits on a healthy track. A little positive self-talk and a few tweaks to your to-do list can make all the difference:

State the positive. Thoughts are self-fulfilling prophecies. Tell yourself, "I can lose weight." "I will get out for my walk today." "I can resist the pastry."

Eat breakfast. Study after study shows that people who lose weight and keep it off eat breakfast every day. Skip this meal and not only do you feel starving by lunchtime, your body thinks it's starving and slows down metabolism to conserve calories.

Keep a food diary for one week. Jotting down everything you eat helps you identify your dietary downfalls, keeps you honest, and makes you think twice before grabbing that second slice of pie.

Hang around fit, healthy people. One major study that followed a group of people for more than 30 years found that a person's risk of obesity increased 57 percent if they had a friend who became obese, and 37 percent if their spouse became obese. (If your spouse is overweight, hit the walking trail together!)

Have one less cookie a day. Or consume one less can of regular soda, or one less glass of orange juice, or three fewer bites of a fast-food hamburger. Doing any of these saves you about 100 calories a day, enough to prevent you from gaining the 1.8 to 2 pounds most people pack on each year.

Join a weight-loss group. The studies are unequivocal: People who attend support groups as part of a comprehensive weight-loss program lose more weight than those who go it alone.

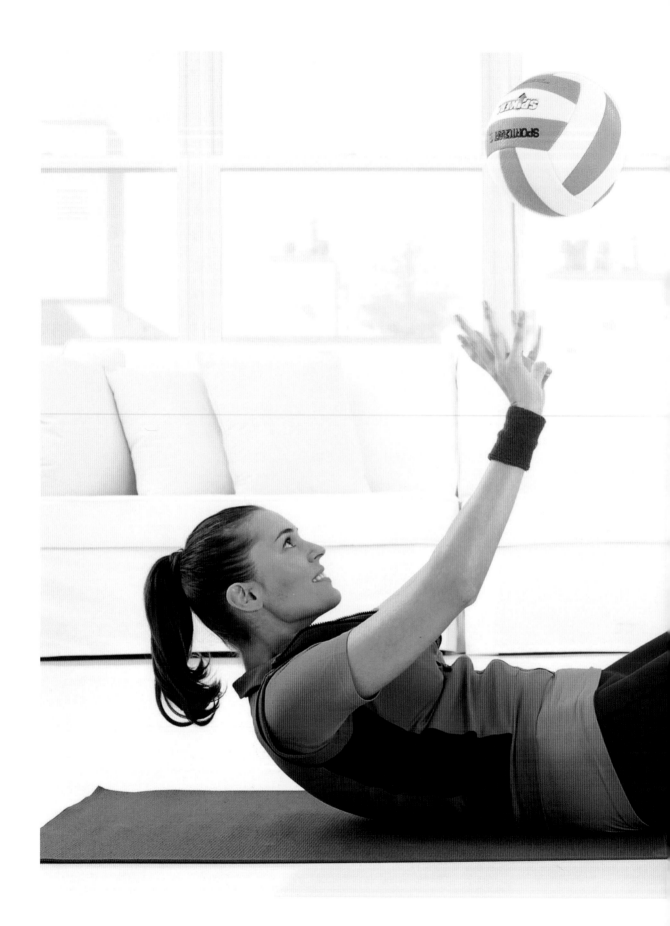

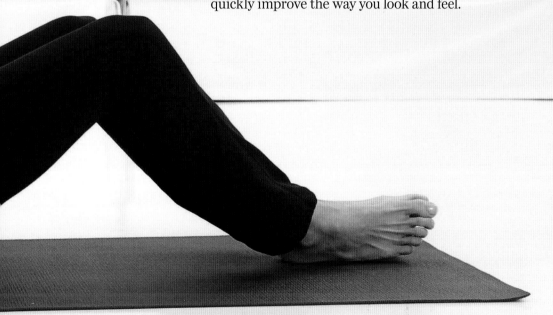

Get Fit
to Walk It Off

IT DOESN'T TAKE LONG to begin to enjoy the benefits of walking. Within days you will feel more energy and more focus, and within weeks you'll start to see that needle moving on your scale.

Incorporating ways to make your entire day a little more active, along with adding some stretching, strength training, and a few simple exercises to boost your flexibility, will quickly improve the way you look and feel.

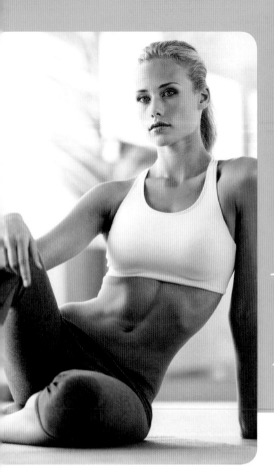

Boost Your *Metabolism* All Day Long

By now you know that fitness and lasting weight loss are better achieved by incorporating movement throughout your day, not just in concentrated bursts at the gym. Take Angelina and Cindy. Angelina works out hard for an hour every day but then spends 90 minutes round-trip commuting by car, 8 hours working at a computer, and the rest of the evening watching Netflix. Meanwhile, Cindy doesn't exercise per se, but she's active all day long doing housework, gardening, and running errands.

So who is more fit, healthy, and burns more calories? Researchers in the department of exercise science at the University of South Carolina recently did this comparison (although their subjects weren't named Angelina or Cindy), and their conclusion may surprise you.

Most trainers and doctors classify anyone who gets 30 to 60 minutes of moderate to vigorous daily exercise (like Angelina) as "active." Anyone who doesn't (like Cindy) is considered "sedentary." But when you dig into Angelina's lifestyle, you find that her 7 total hours of weekly exercise constitute just 5 percent of her week. That means she's inactive 95 percent of the time. If Cindy engages in light activity 75 percent of each day, researchers determined that she actually uses about 10 percent more energy than Angelina. And if you equate energy expenditure with being fit, healthy, and lean, then maybe our whole approach to exercise needs some rethinking.

"When we started researching exercise some 30 years ago, the focus was on vigorous activity," says Russell Pate, PhD, the USC professor who led the investigation. "Then we looked at moderate activity. Now we're dropping down even more and examining light activity and its potential health benefits…. We should probably no longer assume that being sedentary and being active are the inverse of one another."

It's hard to imagine how scurrying around doing errands all day trumps a dedicated hour-long sweat. The fact is, our society has become so automated in the last few decades (even car doors now close by themselves) that we're moving less and less. Such prolonged periods of dormancy may be reaching the point where they're actually offsetting some of the benefits of going to the gym or taking dedicated walks. How? By slowing down the body's metabolism. The hotter and longer your body's furnace runs, the more fuel, or calories, it burns. Although a good workout or brisk walk certainly stokes the furnace, doing nothing for long periods cools it off. It's the sum of your activity—those 10,000 steps a day you're aiming for—and metabolism that determines your total energy expenditure and, ultimately, how you look in your swimsuit this summer.

What Does It Take?

So exactly how much lifestyle activity is required to keep your metabolic furnace lit and you lean?

James A. Levine, MD, a professor of medicine at the Mayo Clinic, has conducted some groundbreaking research into what he's termed non-exercise activity thermogenesis, or NEAT. In plain English this is the amount of energy you use during the normal course of your day, excluding time in the gym or dedicated walking. To measure it, he actually built motion-sensing underwear (take that, Victoria's Secret!) to track subjects' every move. And he found that the difference between people who are overweight and those who aren't is 150 minutes, or 2½ hours, of puttering around each day. That's roughly equivalent to burning 350 calories, or a pint of ice cream.

"It's not uncommon for people to spend half of their waking day sitting," explains Marc Hamilton, PhD, an associate professor of biomedical sciences at the University of Missouri. And just as an idle computer dims to save power, your body starts to shut down at the cellular level when you sit for prolonged periods, barely using large hip and leg muscles. What's more, limiting simple activities like standing and strolling slows down and eventually switches off key fat-burning enzymes such as lipoprotein lipase (LPL), responsible for breaking down

MOST TRAINERS AND DOCTORS CLASSIFY ANYONE WHO GETS 30 TO 60 MINUTES OF MODERATE TO VIGOROUS DAILY EXERCISE AS ACTIVE.

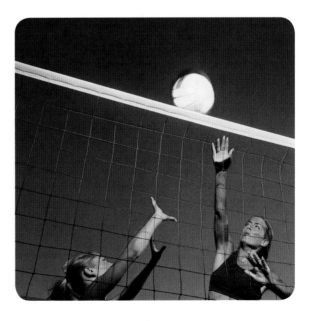

triglycerides in the blood. Sit for a full day and the activity of these fat-burners plummets by 50 percent. Surprisingly, vigorous exercise doesn't seem to turn them back on as well as simply moving around.

In an Australian study, researchers monitoring 168 men and women reported that those who took more breaks from sitting had slimmer waistlines, lower BMIs, healthier blood sugar levels, and better triglyceride and cholesterol profiles than those who sat continuously. And this was despite how much (or how little) moderate-to-vigorous exercise they did otherwise.

Little Ways to Boost Metabolism and Drop Pounds

LEAN PEOPLE SPEND AN AVERAGE OF 150 MINUTES OF NON-EXERCISE TIME STANDING, MOVING, FIDGETING, AND PUTTERING EVERY DAY.

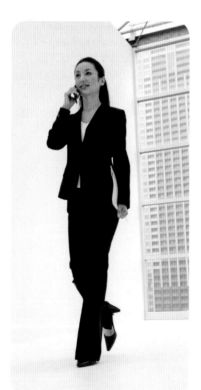

In addition to all the obvious tricks, such as taking the stairs instead of the elevator, parking farther away from your destination, and washing the car by hand, try these strategies for building more movement into your day.

Walk while talking. Make a rule for yourself: Every time you're on the phone, walk around while talking (or pace back and forth if you're limited by a cord). Squeezing in 5 to 10 minutes of movement has never been easier.

Talk instead of e-mailing. Experts at the Stanford Prevention Research Center found that spending 2 minutes e-mailing a colleague rather than walking down the hall to speak with them resulted in a 10-pound weight gain over 10 years. Yikes! Delete!

Lift while watching. If you enjoy watching *The View* in the morning, keep a dumbbell handy and do 10 biceps curls whenever one of them takes a sip of coffee. The possibilities for small movements are endless.

Wear a pedometer all day. Instead of using it as you usually do (to track total daily steps), divide your activity-level monitoring into two separate parts: during your walk and during the rest of your day. The results may surprise you. If it turns out you're taking most of your daily steps during your workout, then your lifestyle is imbalanced and it could be thwarting your attempts at fitness and weight loss. As we've seen, it's better to distribute movement more equitably throughout the day. We're not suggesting that you abandon your dedicated exercise session. It still holds important cardiovascular, fat-burning, and fitness benefits. Rather, the key is adding more movement to your day *outside* of your dedicated walks to keep your metabolism humming.

Suck in your gut. Tightening your abdominal muscles for 60 seconds at a time when you're standing, driving your car, or sitting at your desk or the

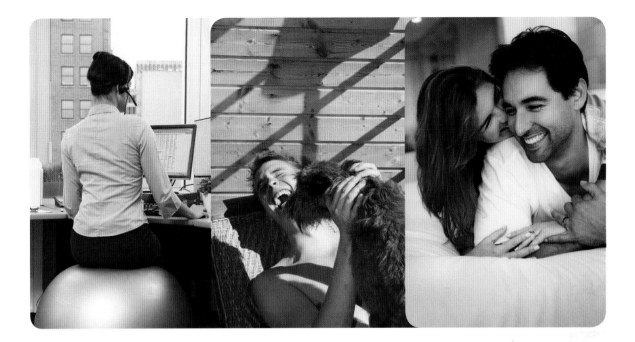

dinner table will build strength in your core, which in turn improves posture and burns fat to flatten that belly.

Trade your chair for a ball. Swapping your desk chair for an exercise ball will help you be more active while sitting at the computer by recruiting muscles in your legs and torso to maintain your balance.

Use a smaller mug at work. Or a smaller water bottle. The result: more trips to the coffee machine or watercooler.

Track your calories. Besides pedometers, new devices—like the bodybugg (www.bodybugg.com) FitBit (www.fitbit.com), and Nike+Sportband (www.nike.com)—track calories burned in addition to steps taken, supplying an additional level of assessment and motivation.

Squeeze your butt cheeks. A great way to a great butt! Do it in your car or at your desk! No one needs to know.

Try twice-a-day workouts. If your job or lifestyle is such that you can't be getting up and moving around a lot, then split your exercise time into two smaller parts. For instance, if you're used to taking an hour-long walk in the evening after work, switch to a half hour over lunch and a half hour after dinner. Two bouts of shorter exercise like this will keep your metabolism revving higher than one longer one.

Love more. Did you know that having sex three times a week—don't worry, nothing fancy—burns 7,500 calories per year, which is equivalent to jogging 75 miles?

TO LOSE WEIGHT AND KEEP IT OFF FOR GOOD, TAKE EXERCISE OUT OF THE GYM AND SPREAD IT THROUGH-OUT YOUR DAY.

TAKE 10

Feeling overwhelmed, overextended, and just plain out of time? Even if it will make you late for the next item on your jam-packed schedule, take a 10-minute walk to catch your breath, calm your anxiety, and clear your head. Concentrate on your breathing--not about the next thing on your to-do list—and keep a strong but relaxed posture. Pay attention to the details of your surroundings (Hey, that lilac bush is in bloom! Did the people who live in the house on the corner get a new car?) to get your head in another place. One walker we know likes to belt out a Broadway tune or two to get her day back on track.

This short walk will help you regain your balance and make better decisions about how you use your time.

Laugh more. It's estimated that 100 belly laughs delivers an aerobic workout similar to 10 minutes on a rowing machine. Take a break during your day for a funny and you'll boost your metabolism.

Stand while working. Most of us don't have a fancy standing desk with a treadmill in front of it (though that would be one great way to stay awake while working). But if you have a laptop and high shelf or, at home, a tall dresser, place your laptop where you can stand while working, if only for 10 minutes at a time. Your lower back will thank you, and you'll burn calories while barely moving.

Fidget more. Shake your foot, bounce your leg, tap your fingers, do heel raises or toe circles at your desk—it all adds up. Studies show that fidgeting burns substantial calories.

Squeeze a stress ball. Even if you're not stressed. You'll burn calories in addition to building stronger forearm muscles. Keep one in your car and use it at red lights.

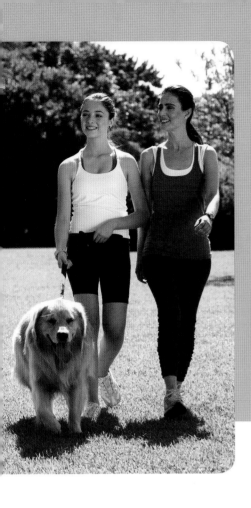

Fine-Tune Your Machine

Walking is to exercise what, say, Frank Stella is to art: spare, minimalist, and elegant in its simplicity. Lace up and head out—that's all we walkers need to do. Bada bing, bada boom. No gym membership required.

But what if a little elaboration—think a Kandinsky-esque flourish here or there—improved your time on the pavement and made walking more pleasant and comfortable? That's exactly what these stretches and strength moves will do. Study after study has proved that regular strength training makes your muscles stronger, boosts endurance, increases tone, and protects you from injury by adding thickness to joint-cushioning connective tissues such as ligaments and preventing bone loss. Stretching increases your range of motion and, well, just feels great.

To add a little (twice-weekly) embellishment to your walking routine, try these toes-to-shoulder stretches and strength moves for walkers. Still no gym membership required.

The muscles of the ankles and feet are small, so simple exercises with only slight resistance are all that's necessary to give them an excellent workout.

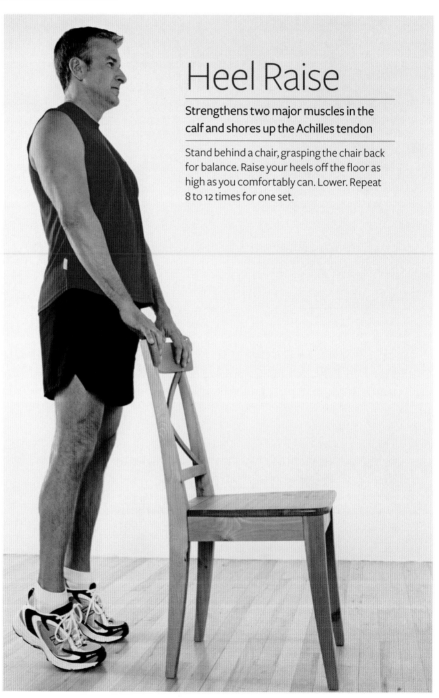

BEFORE OR AFTER: WHEN SHOULD YOU STRETCH?

For years experts believed that stretching before a workout helped prevent exercise-induced injuries. But a pile of recent research suggests otherwise. The new wisdom? It's more important to warm up before exercising (for instance, by strolling for a few minutes before a fitness walk) than to stretch, which can actually cause your muscles to tire more quickly. Save stretching for after your cool-down.

Heel Raise

Strengthens two major muscles in the calf and shores up the Achilles tendon

Stand behind a chair, grasping the chair back for balance. Raise your heels off the floor as high as you comfortably can. Lower. Repeat 8 to 12 times for one set.

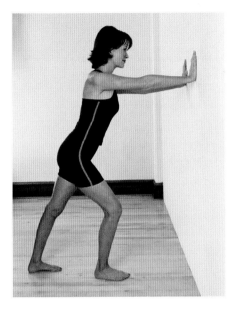

Calf Stretch

Limbers up the calves and stretches the Achilles tendon

Stand about 18 inches (46 cm) from a wall and place your hands on the wall. Take a big step backward with your right foot. Bending your left knee, keep your right leg straight and your right heel flat on the floor to produce a gentle tug at the back of your lower leg. Move your hips forward to increase the stretch. Switch sides and repeat.

Ankle Circle

Promotes ankle mobility

Sit in a chair with your legs extended slightly. Rotate your ankles in a circular motion. Do this 6 to 8 times, then change direction. To work your legs at the same time, elevate your feet.

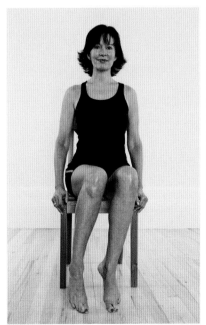

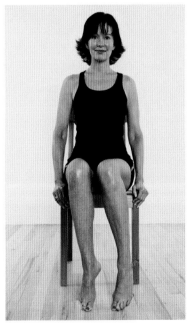

They take the brunt of your walks, so treat 'em right!

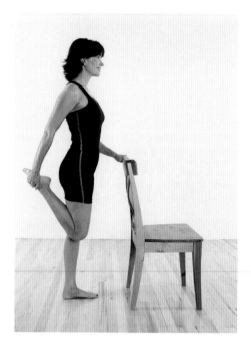

Standing Quad Stretch

Stretches the quadriceps muscle at the front of the thigh

Stand with your feet about hip-width apart, holding on to a chair back with your right hand. Keeping your right knee slightly flexed, grab your left foot with your left hand and gently bring the heel toward your buttocks. Keep your knees aligned. Hold. Release your foot, and repeat with your right.

Knees to Chest

Stretches the lower back, hips, and knees

Lie on your back with your legs straight and relaxed. Place your hands on the backs of your thighs under your knees and pull both knees toward your chest, keeping your lower back on the floor. Hold.

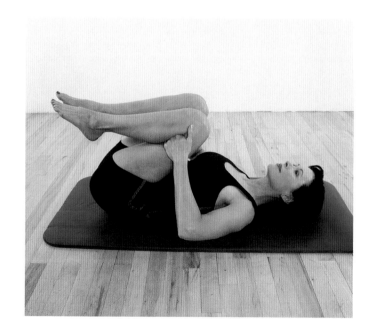

Partial Lunge

Builds the large muscles involved in walking

Holding on to the back of a chair, take a giant step forward with your right foot. Keeping your upper body straight, bend your right knee, and slide your pelvis forward until your knee is over the toe of your right foot. The heel of your left foot will come off the floor. To further lower your body, bend your left knee. Return to the starting position, and repeat 8 to 12 times. Switch sides.

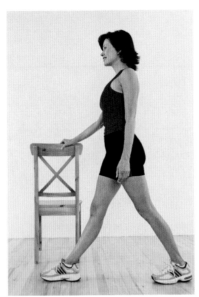
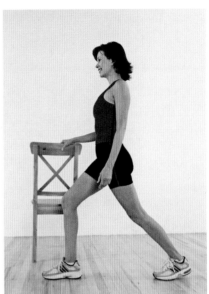

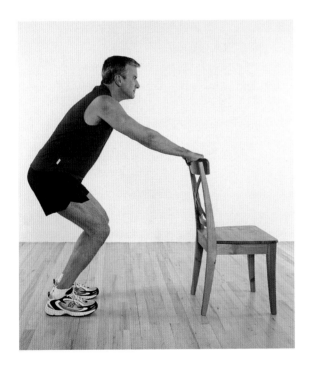

Partial Squat

Builds quadriceps, hamstrings, and buttocks

Stand with your feet hip-width apart, lightly touching a chair back for balance. Keeping your back straight and your eyes looking forward, lower your body as if you were going to sit in a chair. Make sure your knees do not extend beyond your toes. Stop halfway to a sitting position, then raise yourself back up. Repeat 8 to 12 times for one set. To amp it up, lower yourself all the way to the front half of a chair.

Stretch and strengthen the muscles that support the spine—and help prevent back pain.

Superman

Hits muscles from the base of your head to your buttocks, all of which add stability to your spine

Lie on your stomach with your arms extended in front of you and your eyes looking at your hands. Holding your chin off the floor, gently lift your arms and feet off the floor, hold for 1 second, and lower. Repeat 8 to 12 times for one set. If you feel discomfort in your neck, keep your eyes facing the floor and rest your head on a pillow instead of lifting your chin.

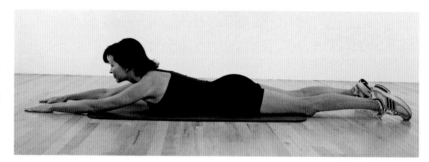

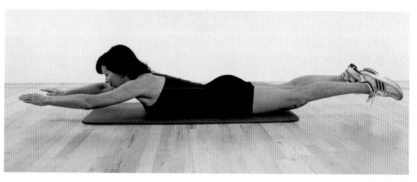

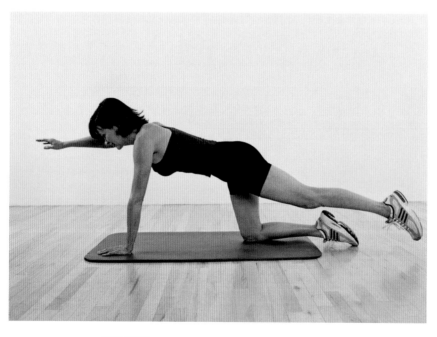

Bird Dog

Works the muscles of the back, hips, and shoulders

Get down on your hands and knees. Keeping your abs tight for support, extend your left leg out behind you so it's parallel to the floor. At the same time, reach in front of you with your right arm. Return to the starting position and repeat with the other leg and arm to complete one repetition. Repeat 8 to 12 times.

Pelvic Twist

A great lower-back stretch

Lie on your back with knees bent, feet flat on the floor, and your arms extended straight out from your sides. Gently lower both knees to your right side until you feel a slight stretch in your left lower-back and hip area. Hold, then return to the starting position. Repeat on the other side.

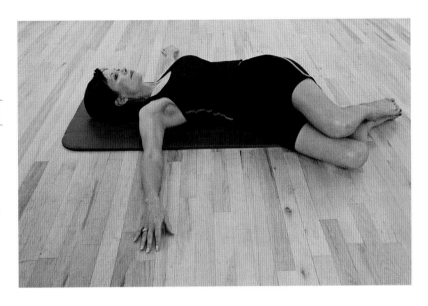

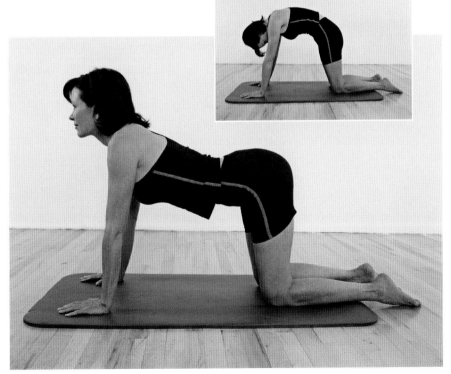

Cat Stretch

A feel-good spine stretch

Get on your hands and knees. Tuck your chin toward your chest and tighten your stomach muscles to arch your back. Hold. Relax, raising your head so that you're looking straight ahead while letting your stomach sink toward the floor. Hold.

Strong abs are critical for good posture because they are key to supporting the muscles in your back, which in turn support your spine. With strong abs you will decrease stress on joints in the neck, hip, knees, and ankles. And you'll reduce the chance of back problems and appear taller, too—even if you don't achieve a six-pack!

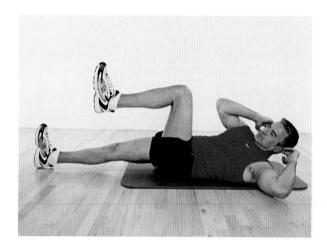

Bicycle

Strengthens the abs and sides

Lie flat on your back with your legs straight and your hands behind your ears. Lift your head off the floor and bring your left knee toward your head, stopping when your thigh is perpendicular to the floor. At the same time, bring your right elbow toward the knee. Return to starting position. Rest for 1 second and repeat on the opposite side. Continue for 30 seconds for one set.

Ball Stretch

Stretches the latticework of muscles throughout your abdomen

With an exercise ball positioned under your upper back, your hips lowered toward the floor, and your knees bent about 90 degrees. Slowly straighten your legs, rolling on your back along the ball, keeping your feet on the floor until you feel a stretch in your abdominal area.

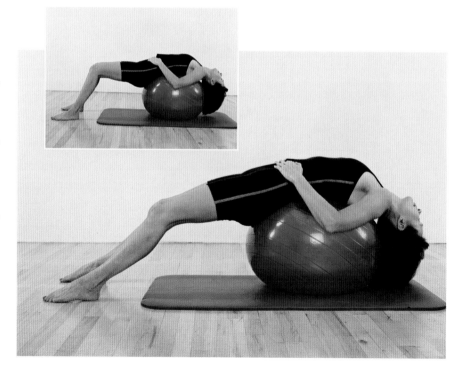

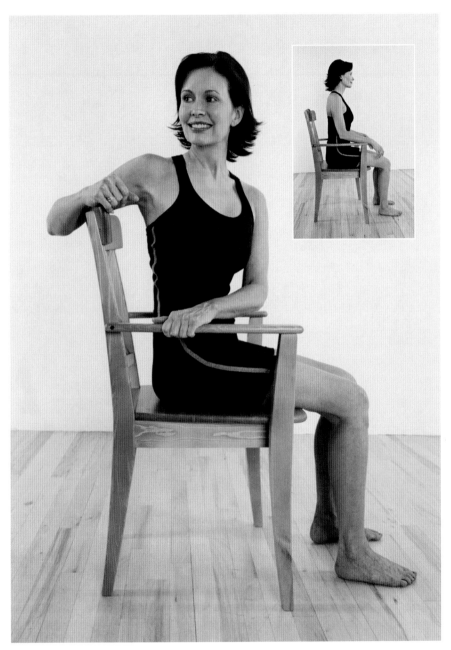

Seated Torso Twist

An anytime stretch for the torso

Sit in a straight-backed chair that has arms, with your feet flat on the floor and your legs bent 90 degrees. Turn your upper body at the waist to the left, grabbing the arm of the chair to assist in the twist, and look over your left shoulder. Relax and hold, breathing normally. Return to the starting position and repeat on the other side.

GET A HARD CORE
Make the most of your walks—even casual strolls through parking lots—by strengthening your core while you amble. Simply draw your abdominal muscles in as far as you can and hold for 5 seconds. Let your gut out and repeat. It's like doing crunches on the run.

Your chest muscles are also important in helping you maintain good posture and are responsible for supporting the movement of your arms and shoulders.

Wall Push-Up

Less challenging than a regular push-up but still effective

From a standing position about 18 inches from a wall, put your hands on the wall about shoulder-width apart at chest level, with your palms flat and fingers pointed toward the ceiling. Slowly lower your chin toward the wall, keeping your elbows out to the side. Smoothly push back from the wall to the starting position. Repeat 8 to 12 times.

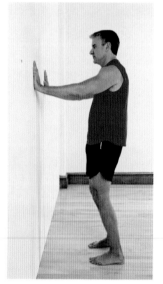
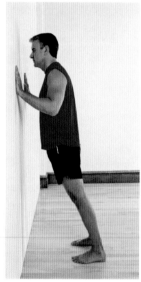

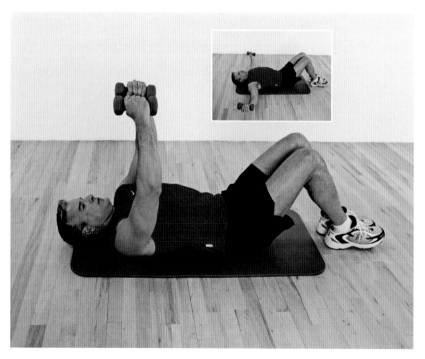

Weighted Chest Fly

Works the chest and arms and helps stabilize the shoulder joints

Lie on your back with your knees bent and feet flat on the floor, light hand weights on either side of you. Grab the weights and press them toward the ceiling, your palms facing each other. This is your starting position. Maintaining a slight bend in your elbows, inhale as you extend your arms out from your sides until they're a few inches from the floor. Exhale as you press your hands back up to the starting position. Repeat 8 to 12 times for one set.

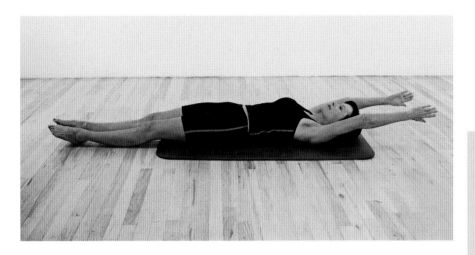

Lying Total Body Stretch

Stretches the chest and abdomen

Lie on your back on a mat with your legs extended. Extend your arms straight over your head and stretch your legs and toes, making your entire body as long as comfortably possible. Hold.

ARE YOU POSTURE PERFECT?

Maintaining good posture while walking is important for balance, avoiding injury, and getting the most fat-burning bang for your buck when you walk. Good posture throughout the rest of the day can help you breathe properly, which sends more oxygen to your brain, increasing your ability to concentrate and think critically.

Wall Stretch

Lengthens the same muscles as the wall push-up

Stand with your feet together and your left side next to a wall. Take one step forward with your right foot. Place your left forearm vertically against the wall with your elbow bent at 90 degrees so your upper arm is parallel to the floor. Keeping your back heel flat on the floor, bend your right knee so that your body moves forward and you feel a stretch in your chest and upper arm. Hold and repeat on the other side.

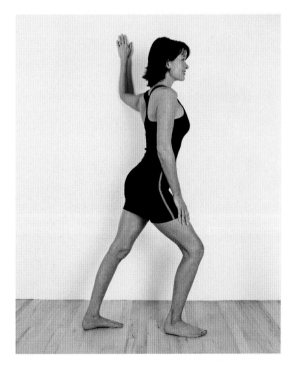

arms and shoulders

Your legs aren't the only things that swing when you walk. Power up your arm swing by strengthening your arms and shoulders.

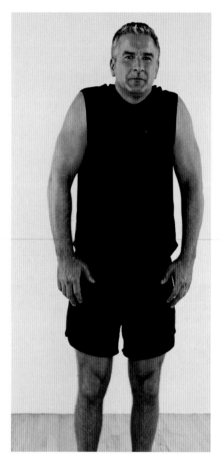

Shoulder Roll

Helpful if you have tension in your neck or upper back

Move your shoulders forward to stretch your shoulder blades, then raise them toward your ears. Now move them backward so the shoulder blades squeeze together. Relax. Repeat 6 times.

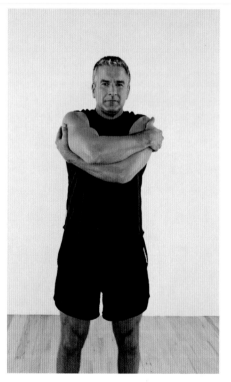

Self-Hug

Stretches the back of the shoulders

Wrap your arms around yourself, reaching each hand to grasp the opposite shoulder to produce a stretch in the back of the shoulders. Hold.

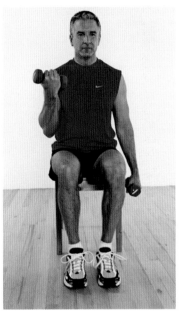
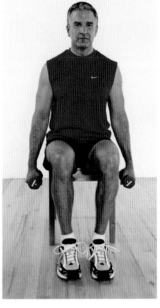

Biceps Curl

The classic biceps toner

Sit up straight on the front half of an armless chair with your feet flat on the floor, your arms by your sides, and a hand weight in each hand. Keeping your elbow at your side, raise the weight in your right hand toward your shoulder while rotating your palm a quarter turn so it faces your shoulder at the top of the movement. Slowly return to the starting position and repeat with the left arm for one repetition. Repeat 8 to 12 times for one set.

Triceps Kickback

Works the muscles at the back of your upper arms

Stand in front of a chair holding a hand weight in your left hand. Bend forward at the waist, putting your right hand on the chair. Keeping your knees slightly bent, bring the weight to your rib cage. This is your starting position. Keeping your elbow next to your body, 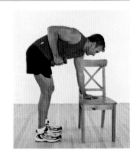 smoothly push the weight behind you, extending your elbow until it is nearly straight. Hold for 1 second and slowly lower the weight to the starting position. Repeat 8 to 12 times for one set. Repeat with the right arm.

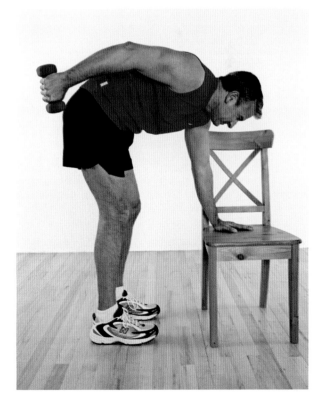

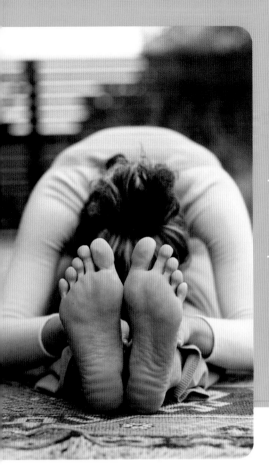

Aim to Be *Flexible*

Strength training ups the ante for walkers, to be sure. But walkers can also get big bonus benefits from improving flexibility, too. Smart stretching aimed at increasing flexibility is good for any body; it leaves you feeling loose, relaxed, and stress-free. It's especially good for walkers because it concentrates your flexibility in hard-to-stretch but often sore spots, like your neck, feet, hips, and back. You can do this routine any time you feel the need to stretch out, but it's best done after walking to keep your body from tightening up and to ensure that you are ready to roll again the next day.

Hold each stretch for 30 to 60 seconds unless otherwise indicated.

Extended Triangle

Stretches your upper legs, abs, back, and sides

Start with your feet wide apart in a straddle stance. Raise your arms out to the sides, parallel to the floor, palms facing down. Turn your left foot out 90 degrees. Keeping your arms extended, bend from the hip and extend your torso to the left directly over your left leg. Rest your left hand on top of your left foot (or on your ankle or shin if you can't reach) while reaching toward the ceiling with your right hand, palm forward. Turn your head to gaze up toward your right hand. Hold for 30 seconds. Switch sides.

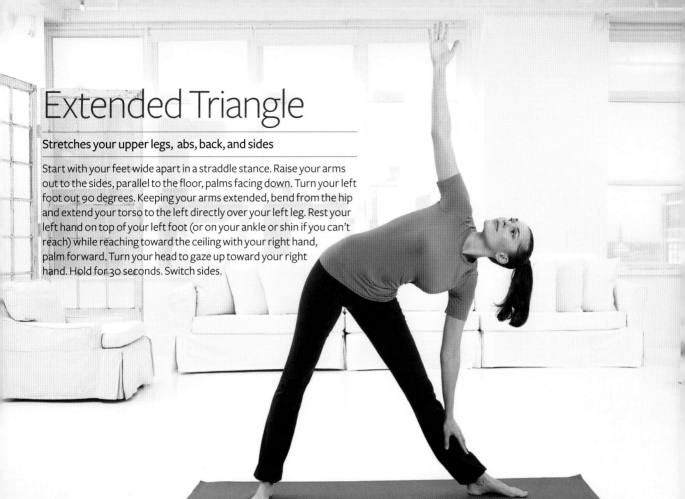

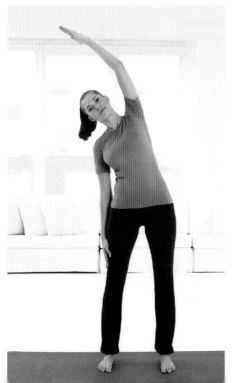

Sky Reach & Bend

Stretches sides, shoulders, arms, back, and hips

Stand with your feet hip-width apart, arms at your sides, palms facing in. Extend your left arm straight up from your side, reaching over your head to the opposite side as far as comfortably possible, keeping your shoulders down and relaxed. Hold for 30 seconds. Repeat to the other side.

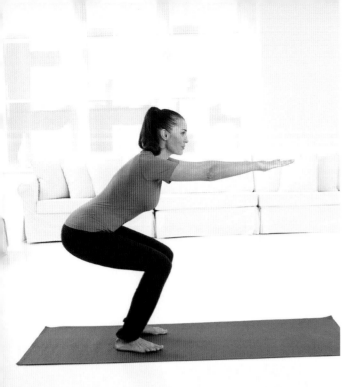

Sit Back

Stretches back, sides, and hips

Stand tall with your feet close together, shoulders back. Raise your arms straight out in front of you, palms down. Bend your knees and sit back, trying to lower your thighs as close to parallel with the ground as possible, allowing your torso to lean slightly forward over your thighs. Keep your back long and straight as you hold the stretch. Then straighten your knees and lower your arms to return to a stand.

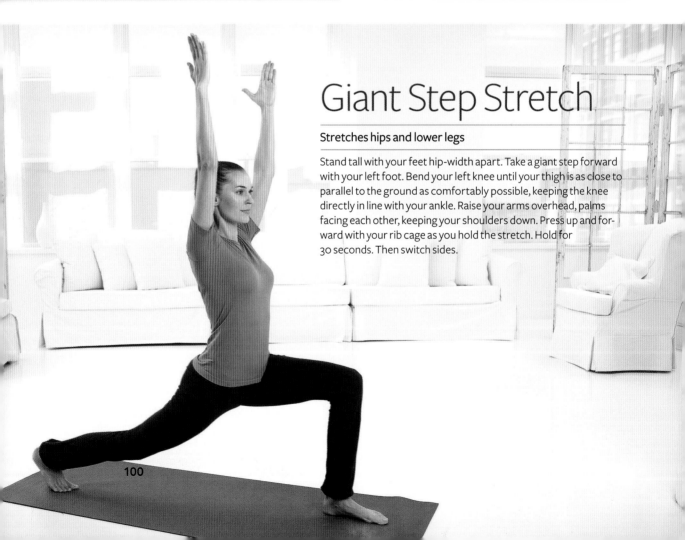

Giant Step Stretch

Stretches hips and lower legs

Stand tall with your feet hip-width apart. Take a giant step forward with your left foot. Bend your left knee until your thigh is as close to parallel to the ground as comfortably possible, keeping the knee directly in line with your ankle. Raise your arms overhead, palms facing each other, keeping your shoulders down. Press up and forward with your rib cage as you hold the stretch. Hold for 30 seconds. Then switch sides.

Rag Doll to Open Arms

Stretches back, shoulders, chest, arms, and neck

Sit on the edge of a chair and slump your body forward over your legs so your chest rests on your knees and your arms hang down (right). Wrap your arms under your knees and arch your back toward the ceiling (your chest will lift off of your legs). Hold for 30 seconds. Then come back to a seated position, open your knees, and tilt your pelvis slightly forward. Lift your chest and squeeze your shoulder blades together and down away from your ears (below). Extend your arms out from your body at 45-degree angles and reach them slightly behind you, palms facing forward. Hold for 30 seconds.

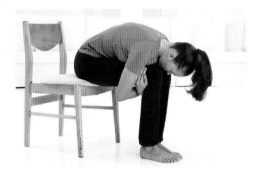

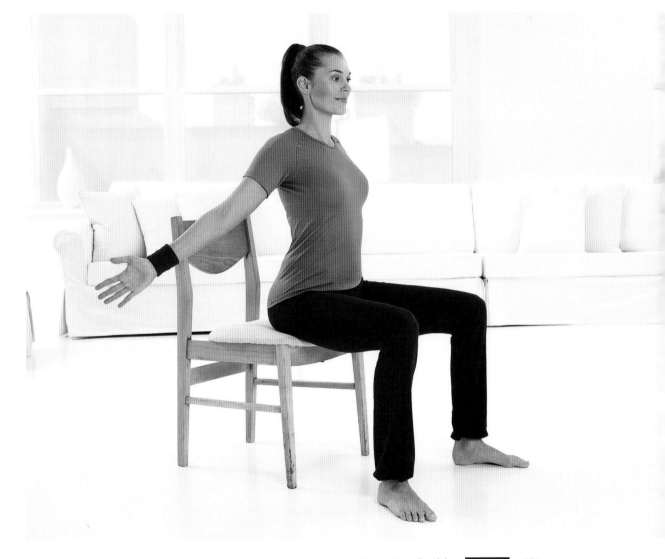

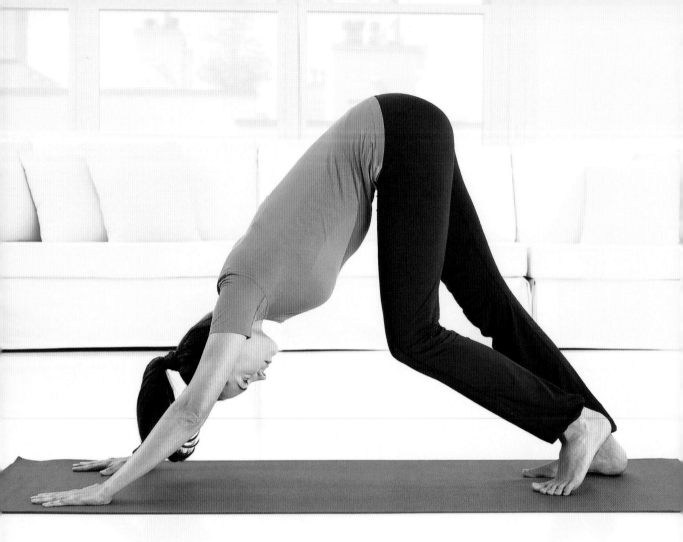

Downward Dog
with Knee Drop

Stretches legs, shoulders, back, and hips

Begin on your hands and knees with your feet hip-width apart, hands directly beneath your shoulders. Press into your palms and straighten your legs, lifting your tailbone toward the ceiling while pulling your navel toward your spine so your body forms an inverted V. Gently press your torso through your arms and your heels toward the floor. Hold for 30 seconds. Next begin "pedaling" your legs: Bend the left knee slightly while extending your right leg, pressing the right heel into the floor. Then switch legs, bending the right knee and extending the left leg. Continue alternating for another 30 seconds.

Scorpion

Stretches back, hips, and core

Lie facedown with your arms out to the sides, shoulders flat on the floor. Lift your right leg off the floor and, twisting your torso, reach it across the back of your body as far as possible toward your left hand. Return to start. Then repeat to the other side. Repeat this motion for 30 to 60 seconds.

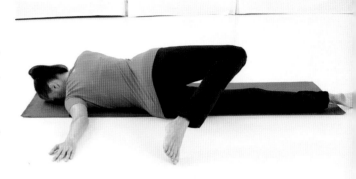

Prayer Pose

Stretches back and shoulders

Kneel with the tops of your feet on the floor, toes pointed behind you. Sit back onto your heels and lower your chest to your thighs. Stretch your arms out overhead and rest your palms and forehead on the floor (or as close as possible).

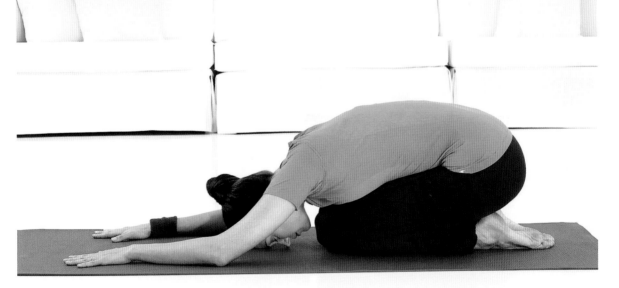

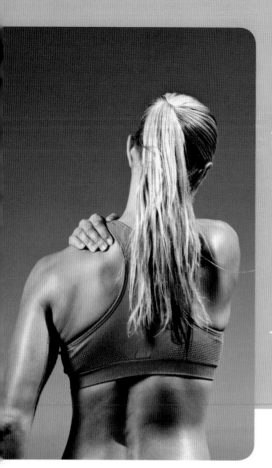

What to Do When It Hurts

You've heard the expression "No pain, no gain." Well, you can forget it. A body that's in pain simply cannot make physical gains. Here's a guide to minimizing some of the most common walking-related complaints so you can feel better fast and keep your gams in the game.

Muscle Soreness

You no doubt know it well: You add a killer hill to your walk or perhaps push yourself to your sweaty best at the gym, and the next day you're so sore and stiff you can barely drag yourself out of bed. While researchers aren't certain what exactly causes "delayed-onset muscle soreness," they suspect it's the result of microscopic tears in your muscles, coupled with the inflammation that follows the tears. The ache Rx? Reduce the inflammation. Here's how.

THE BEST WAY TO BEAT A BLISTER

To drain or not to drain? That is the question. Here's the answer.

Don't pop blisters that are small or unlikely to pop on their own. They're less prone to infection if you leave the natural covering intact, and under the sheltering cushion of fluid, the area has time to form new skin. Simply keep the blister clean with soap and water and cover it with a bandage or a piece of moleskin. To soothe any itching or burning, smear on Preparation H. It works.

If your blister is large or in a spot where you can't avoid putting pressure on it, drain it—but do it the proper way:

Sterilize a needle with rubbing alcohol, and clean the blister the same way. Lay a sterile gauze pad on top of the blister. Pierce the edge of the blister, sliding the needle in sideways, and gently squeeze out the liquid by pressing on the gauze pad. Make sure you don't tear or remove that top layer of skin. Smear on an antibiotic ointment, and cover it with a bandage you change twice a day. If the blister refills again later, drain it the same way.

Finally, to sidestep a blister altogether, cover any friction-prone spots with a lubricant, such as Lube-Stick for Runners, before you go for your walk.

CHILL OUT WITH AN ICE MASSAGE. Freeze an inch or two of water in a paper or Styrofoam cup and peel off the top of the cup to expose the edge of the ice. Grasp the bottom part of the cup and glide the exposed ice over your sore muscle. Massage for up to 20 minutes several times a day if the soreness is less than 48 hours old. After 48 hours switch from ice to heat, applying a heating pad for the same duration and frequency.

AGREE TO AN ANTI-INFLAMMATORY. Don't be a hero. Take ibuprofen (400 to 60 mg) or Aleve (225 mg) throughout the day, following the package instructions, for up to two days after exertion.

GIVE MUSCLES THE RUB. Studies shown that rubbing muscles achy from exertion can significantly reduce soreness later on. To further ease the ache, rub a sports cream like BenGay or a natural product like Tiger Balm or White Flower Oil (available at health-food stores) into the sore area after you massage it.

SOAK UP THE SORENESS. A hot bath will help ease the ache, especially if you add a cup or two of Epsom salt to the tub. As it draws fluid through the skin, Epsom salt also draws out lactic acid, which builds up during exercise and can contribute to muscle aches.

KEEP MOVING. As long as you don't overdo it, staying active works the painful chemical by-products of overexertion out of your muscles and keeps the muscle fibers flexible so they won't tighten up further and stay sore longer. Try working the parts of your body that aren't as sore. For instance, if your quads ache from climbing hills, walk a flat course or, better yet, hit the pool for a swim.

FIGHT MUSCLE CRAMPS BEFORE 9 A.M.

Low levels of potassium, calcium, and magnesium—minerals known as electrolytes that help maintain proper fluid balance in your body and are critical to muscle function—can raise your odds of having sudden, painful muscle cramps. Get more of all three by eating a bowl of whole-grain cereal with milk and sliced bananas at breakfast and popping a multivitamin. Also, drink plenty of water throughout the day, since cramping can also be a sign of dehydration.

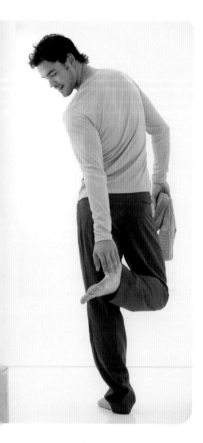

Foot Pain

Sometimes foot pain has an obvious cause—a corn, callus, or ingrown toenail. But if your trotters are howling due to plain old pavement pounding, you may need a foot doctor less than you need some tootsy TLC. The ache Rx? Pamper your feet. Here's how:

SOAK YOUR SIZE 8s. For a refreshing and stimulating treat for the feet, fill one basin with cold water and another with water as hot as you can comfortably stand. Sit in a chair in front of the basins, and place your feet in the cold water. After 5 minutes switch to the hot water. Repeat. This "hydromassage" alternately dilates and constricts blood vessels in your feet, boosting circulation.

An alternate tack: Fill a basin with hot water and add two drops of peppermint oil, along with four drops each of eucalyptus and rosemary oil. Soak for 10 minutes. If you don't have any essential oils at home, brew a very strong cup of peppermint tea and add it to the water.

ROLL THE PAIN AWAY. In health-food stores you can buy a roller specially designed to massage the soles of the feet. Or you can simply roll your bare foot over a tennis ball, golf ball, or rolling pin for several minutes. You can also borrow this trick from the fancy spas. Get a couple of smooth stones around the size of the palm of your hand. Soak them in hot water until they're nice and warm, then place them in a plastic basin and run the balls, then the arches, then the heels slowly over the stones.

GIVE YOUR FEET A WORKOUT. Scatter a few pencils on the floor and pick them up with your toes. This exercise helps relieve foot pain. Or wrap a thick rubber band around all the toes on one foot. Spread your toes and hold for 5 seconds. Repeat 10 times to relieve the ache in shoe-bound feet.

S-T-R-E-T-C-H. Heel pain, especially in the morning, may signal plantar fasciitis, an inflammation of the tough band of tissue that connects your heel bone to the base of your toes. To get relief, stretch your Achilles tendon. Stand about 3 feet from a wall. Place your hands on the wall, and move your right leg forward, knee bent. Keep your left leg straight, with your heel on the floor. You should feel a gentle stretch in your heel and foot arch. Hold for 10 seconds, then switch sides and repeat. If the pain is bad, see your doctor, who might prescribe a splint to keep your foot flexed when you sleep.

SHOULD I DIAL MY DOC?

Occasionally aching feet are nothing to worry about; persistent foot pain, however, is a matter for an MD. See a podiatrist or orthopedic surgeon specializing in feet if you find it hard to walk first thing in the morning or if the painful area is swollen or discolored. You may have a broken bone, inflamed tendon, or pinched nerve. Ditto if there's a painful burning sensation in your feet, which may indicate diabetes or thyroid disease. If you've already been diagnosed with diabetes, see your doc at once if a cut, sore, blister, or bruise on your foot doesn't start to heal after one day.

Shin Splints

If you walk or run regularly, there's a chance you'll develop shin splints. During exercise muscles in the lower leg swell and press against the gap formed by the tibia and fibula, the bones that extend from the knee to the ankle. This pressure irritates nearby muscles, tendons, or ligaments, causing pain along the outer calf (anterior shin splints) or inner calf (posterior shin splints). Posterior shin splints are common among people with flat feet, because the leg muscles have to work hard to support the foot's arch.

The ache Rx? Reduce inflammation with ice, ibuprofen, and rest—and perhaps new walking shoes. Here's how.

STRETCH IT OUT. Sit on the floor with your legs extended in front of you, keeping the painful leg slightly bent. Loop a towel around the ball of your foot and, with the knee still bent, gently pull the towel toward your body. Hold for 15 to 30 seconds, then relax. Repeat three times.

As a follow-up, stand and place your hands against the wall at eye level. Keep your painful shin back, with the heel on the floor, and the good shin forward. Turn your back foot slightly inward, as if pigeon-toed. Slowly lean into the wall until you feel a stretch in the back of your calf. Hold for 15 to 30 seconds.

MAKE SURE YOUR SHOES WORK FOR YOU. Shop for walking shoes at a walking or running specialty store, where the clerks are experts on feet and fit. For instance, if you roll your feet inward (this is called pronation) when you walk, you force your tendons to compensate, increasing your risk of shin splints. You need shoes designed to correct for that tendency.

NUMB THE PAIN. Ice the achy shin to bring down swelling and dull the pain. Either apply a flexible ice pack or bag of frozen vegetables to the shin for 20 minutes (to make sure you don't get frostbite, place a paper towel between the pack and your skin) or perform ice massage (see "Chill Out with Ice Massage" on page 105).

SHOULD I DIAL MY DOC?

You can usually treat shin splints on your own. But if the pain lingers for more than three weeks, give your doctor a call. You may have a stress fracture, a tiny crack in the bone that causes pain in the shinbone and can get much worse without treatment. To diagnose a stress fracture, your doctor will probably order an X-ray, MRI, or bone scan.

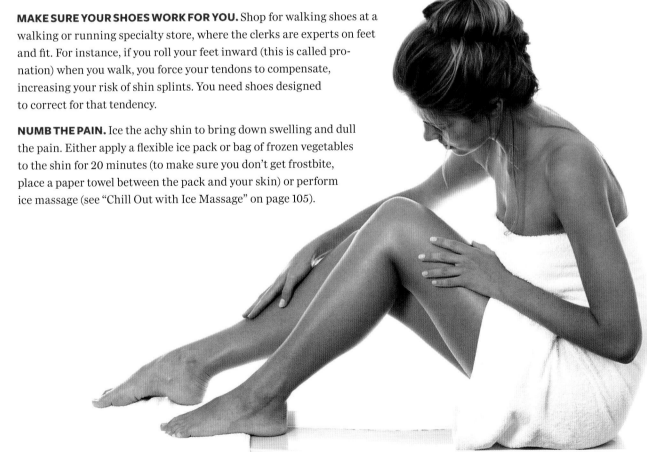

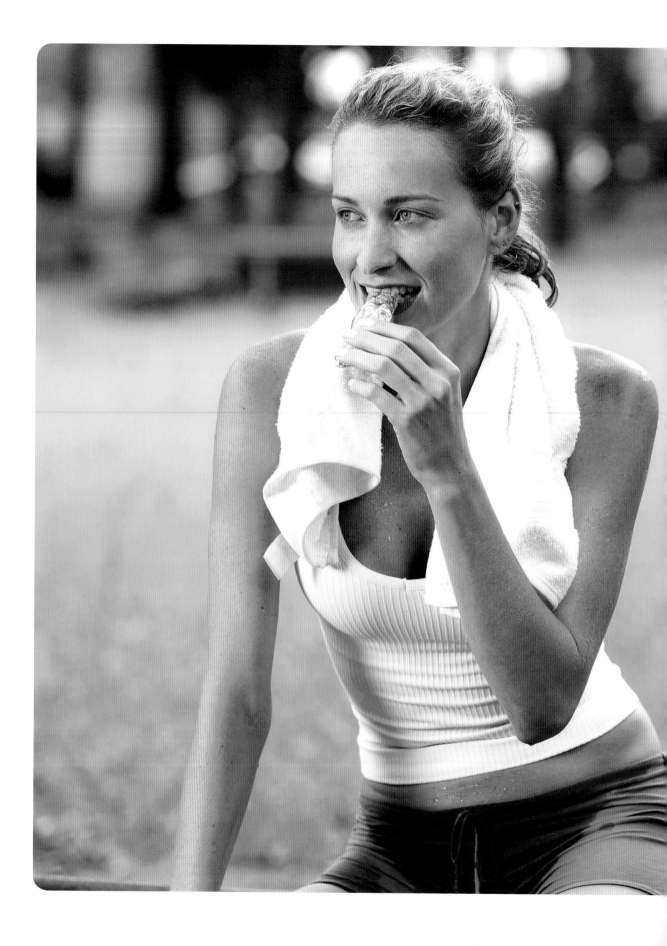

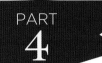

Eat Well
to Walk It Off

THE FOOD PART OF THE WALK IT OFF STRATEGY isn't a diet, but it is about *your* diet. We've learned much in the last 10 years about certain foods and ingredients that deliver powerful benefits related to heart health, weight loss, increased energy, and even improved mental focus. Smart folks are finding ways to include more of these superstar foods in their daily diets, while bumping processed foods, white bread and pasta, and high-sugar stuff off the menu. Changing up what's in your daily diet even just a little can make a big difference. So can changing *how* you eat (for example, downsizing portions or eating more slowly) and the way you deal with cravings versus genuine hunger. Combine a smarter approach to eating with your walking program, and you'll quickly be on your way to a new you.

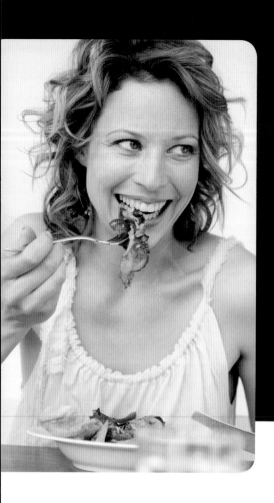

Change the Way You Eat

Say good-bye to the food pyramid and say hello to the "plate." For almost 20 years the U.S. Department of Agriculture's guidelines for healthy eating were illustrated according to a tiered pyramid that identified recommended intake for each food group, measured by the number of servings of each it suggested we should consume. In 2011 the USDA rolled out the "My Plate" program, which depicts the food groups arranged on a plate, indicating an ideal balance of 30 percent grains, 30 percent vegetables, 20 percent fruits, and 20 percent protein, along with a small cup-size circle suggesting a small serving of dairy.

Besides being easier to visualize how the current dietary guidelines apply to our daily lives, the new Food Guide Plate eliminates the need to keep track of numbers of servings or to figure out how large a serving is. Now that we can actually see what a healthy combination of foods looks like, along with correct portion sizes, we should be all set, right? Not quite. Eating smarter is not just about *controlling* what you eat, but developing a whole new mind-set toward food in general and breaking some of the habits that hold you back.

Small Changes Make a Big Difference

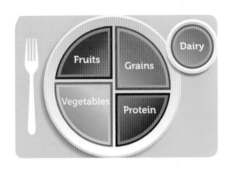

Suppose, just suppose, it's not your food choices that are making you fat but rather *how* you eat. In other words, the speed at which you eat, the type of dinnerware you use, the décor in your dining room, even your dinner companions. Imagine losing 2 or more pounds per month, 12 or more pounds by peak beach season, and 24 or more pounds in a year by making no other changes to your diet than modifying these seemingly superficial factors.

Impossible? Not at all.

Did you know that our brains register fullness about 20 minutes *after* our stomachs do? This lag time causes overeating and, ultimately, weight gain. So here's the simple solution: Make a few easy changes to your eating style, and you will slow down your swallowing and enable your brain to catch up to your belly. As a result, you'll consume fewer calories without feeling any less satisfied. Plus, you'll be able to continue to enjoy your favorite foods because you'll be less apt to overindulge.

Here are 10 scientifically based adjustments that will help you slow down and eat more thoughtfully.

THE USDA'S MYPLATE (CHOOSEMYPLATE.GOV) SHOWS THE PROPORTIONATE AMOUNTS OF EACH FOOD GROUP WE SHOULD CONSUME AT EACH MEAL.

Schedule more time for eating.

Seems contradictory to someone trying to lose weight, doesn't it? But if you allot only a short time to eat, you'll gobble your food down so fast, your body will never have a chance to tell you that you really didn't need so much. So adjust your schedule so you eat your food slowly and calmly over a span of 30 minutes. Two-thirds of the way through, you'll probably start feeling full and lose your desire to continue.

Rest utensils between bites.

This is one of the best ways to stretch your meal out: Make it a personal rule never to have a spoon or fork in your hand while there's food in your mouth. Take a bite, put down the utensil, chew, swallow, then pick it up again and repeat the process.

Substitute chopsticks.

This is another way to guarantee a slow pace. Start by buying a really nice pair that you'd be happy to eat with frequently. Then eat even non-Asian meals with them. Chopsticks pick up much less food with each bite than a fork. They also require more dexterity and concentration. If you find that chopsticks are just too frustrating, try holding your fork or spoon in your nondominant hand.

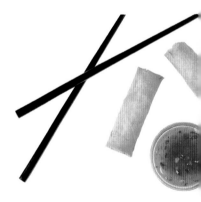

Keep your focus.

Okay, most people prefer company when eating, and if you have a family, you probably insist on it. Doing so provides all kinds of health benefits that have nothing to do

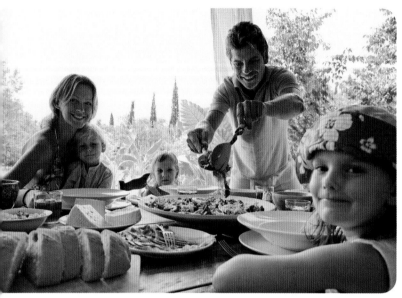

with nutrition. But if you do eat with others, just don't get so lost in conversation that you lose awareness of the eating process. It's important to cherish each bite, eating slowly and mindfully, even while deeply interacting with table mates.

Chew more.

Most of the taste experience actually stems from our sense of smell, which is why nothing tastes good when you have a cold. Use this to your advantage by chewing your food longer. This not only slows down your eating but also allows more of the food's aroma and taste to register. Thus, you'll be less likely to reach for salt, sugar, or other unhealthy flavor enhancers. How much longer should you chew? Brian Wansink, PhD, who runs the Food and Brand Lab at Cornell University, found that normal-weight people chew each bite an average of 15 times, while overweight people chomp 12 times.

Downsize your dinnerware.

Can't resist cream cheese on your bagel or butter on your bread? Use a smaller hors d'oeuvres knife for spreading and you'll tend to use less. Or use a small spoon; study participants given 2-ounce spoons by Dr. Wansink ate 14.5 percent less ice cream than those handed 3-ounce spoons. When a smaller spoon was combined with a smaller bowl, people ate 57 percent less ice cream overall. This strategy holds true for soups, chili, and stews as well.

   Switch to 10-inch (25-cm) plates and 6-inch (15-cm) bowls and you can reduce calorie consumption by about 20 percent and lose nearly 2 pounds per month, according to Dr. Wansink. In a study conducted at an all-you-can-eat Chinese buffet, diners choosing bigger plates took 52 percent more food and ate 45 percent more than those using smaller plates. When Dr. Wansink studied teenagers at a camp cafeteria, those given larger bowls served and consumed 16 percent more cereal than those handed smaller ones.

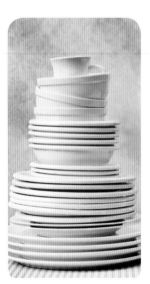

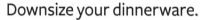

PORTION CONTROL IS EASIER WHEN YOU USE SMALLER DISHES, GLASSES, AND SILVERWARE.

Leave the casserole on the stove.

Easy access to big dishes laden with food is one of the reasons most people overeat at family gatherings. When bowls of food are sitting on the table in front of you, it's just too convenient to extend an arm and dollop out seconds. So whenever you cook large portions, leave the pot or pan in the kitchen rather than setting it on the dining-room table. Provide smaller serving spoons as well. The one exception? Healthily cooked vegetables; strategically placing them within arm's reach will encourage diners to fill up on these low-calorie choices.

Dip forks first.

Instead of slathering your healthful salad with fatty dressing, pour it into a small cup first, then dip your fork and spear some lettuce. This not only reduces your calorie intake (without sacrificing taste), it also puts the brakes on high-speed gobbling.

Drink water between bites.

While water doesn't reduce appetite, it does slow down your eating process. And it's certainly healthy for you. So after every swallow of food, take a small sip of water before picking up your fork again.

Light a vanilla-scented candle.

The aroma has been proven to diminish cravings for sweets.

Kick Your Cravings to the Curb

Let's face it: Half the time, we eat when we aren't even particularly hungry. A host of other needs drive us to the pantry, the fridge, and the vending machine, and if we could only get a handle on those—well, weight problem solved. Fortunately, if you can learn to resist them, you'll watch the pounds drop away!

Ever had an overwhelming craving for a specific food? Or a powerful desire to eat something—anything—salty or sweet? The first craving is a sign that your emotions may be playing a role in your eating habits. The second is a good indication that the food industry has taken over your taste buds, driving you to eat far more food than your body requires in order to get your salt and sugar "fix." Both phenomena make it more difficult to lose weight.

Certain foods even have a direct mood-enhancing effect. Carbohydrates temporarily boost levels of serotonin, a calming, feel-good brain chemical. And eating chocolate and other pleasure-inducing foods triggers the release of endorphins, the chemicals associated with a "runner's high." No wonder we crave them, especially when we're feeling down.

Getting your cravings under control is critical to your weight-loss success. To kick your cravings to the curb once and for all, follow this 5-step plan:

Admit that you're weak.

A big part of the problem with emotional eating is that most women rely on willpower to control it when, as it turns out, they're actually at a disadvantage in this department. A study reported earlier this year from Brookhaven National Laboratory in Upton, New York, found that it's more difficult for women to suppress food cravings than men. Using sophisticated brain scans, researchers detected significantly less activity in the appetite-control centers of women when in the presence of their favorite foods. So forget about using your iron will to resist the cheesecake sitting in front of you. More creative remedies are needed.

STEP 1

Identify your binge buttons.

STEP 2

The best way to do this is to keep a "desire diary." For two weeks write down every craving you have and what you're doing and feeling (stressed, bored, lonely, empty, frustrated) at the time. This will help you pinpoint what's triggering your eating so that you can devise smarter ways to cope. For instance, if you tend to seek out snack food when you first come home from work, you may be eating to alleviate anxiety or pent-up frustration from the day. Instead, try substituting another stress-busting activity, such as taking a short walk or gathering leaves from the yard to use in a centerpiece for the kitchen table.

Likewise, if your diary uncovers a link between feeling lonely and pigging out, then consider asking a friend or family member to be your "craving buddy." When the desire to snack strikes, call or text your lifeline and have her talk you off the Rocky Road. Or surf Facebook instead of cruising the kitchen for food.

Shop and store smarter.

STEP 3

FOOD CRAVINGS ARE NOT THE SAME AS REAL HUNGER. KNOWING THE DIFFERENCE CAN HELP CURB EMPTY SNACKING.

You've heard of putting psychiatric patients in padded rooms so they can't hurt themselves, right? Well, you need to treat your sometimes-crazy eating habits the same way by making your home a crave-free zone. Simply stop buying ice cream, potato chips, soda, or doughnuts. Out of sight, out of stomach. Instead, eat something before heading to the grocery store so you won't make hunger-induced impulse buys and instead choose fruits, vegetables, low-fat yogurt, almonds, and high-fiber whole-grain cereals. These make nutritious snacks that will help you keep future cravings at bay. That's because they digest more slowly than most junk foods and stabilize blood-sugar levels. Replace sugary, fast-digesting snacks with these "low-glycemic" foods and you'll find yourself less hungry. (As a rule of thumb, if the protein, fat, and fiber grams together are equal to or greater than the carb grams, it's low glycemic.)

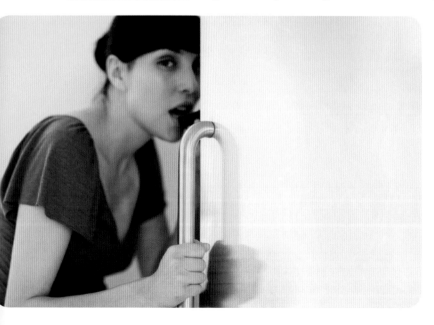

But if your lack of willpower extends even to the supermarket, consider one of these strategies:

Buy the best. If there's one food you absolutely can't resist, then buy the most expensive version of it. Make it hurt. That way, you'll be more inclined to savor it and, in the process, learn portion control. Most times it takes only a small taste of what we're craving to satisfy our urge.

Buy small. It's less environmentally friendly to buy single-serving packages of chips, pretzels, and other snacks, but if you aren't particularly good at exercising self-control, it's a more waist-friendly strategy. So instead of

EMOTIONAL EATERS

Once upon a time, it was enough just for food to fill our bellies. But now we look to food to pick us up when we're sad, help pass the time when we're bored, relax us when we're stressed, and gratify desires when we feel deprived. In other words, we feel compelled to eat at any moment, for any reason. Boss yell at you? Have a candy bar. Late night and feeling lonely? You need some ice cream. Stressful week? A cheeseburger with fries seems the perfect solution.

If we craved spinach or carrots for comfort and joy, there would be no problem. But it's the sweet stuff and the simple starches—mashed potatoes, crackers, chewy white rolls—that many of us desire, and these foods aren't doing our waistlines any favors. Why do we gravitate toward macaroni and cheese instead of, say, green salads? Thank biology. The simple carbohydrates in pasta, crackers, cookies, chips, and French fries trigger the release of serotonin, the same feel-good chemical that some drugs target to get us back on an even emotional keel.

The fix? Try to identify the feelings that make you want to eat when you don't really need to, and find methods to help you control and redirect those impulses away from food.

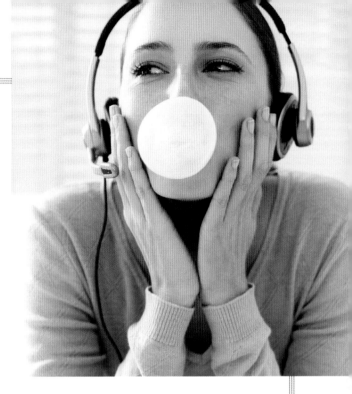

Chew gum.

Sometimes what drives you to the refrigerator is simply a need to move your jaw, and that can be satisfied by a stick of gum. Keep several packs of sugar-free gum around the house and the office so that anytime you feel the urge to eat, you can pop a stick in your mouth.

Relax first; eat second.

When you come home from a long, busy day, chances are you're tempted to eat whatever's in sight. Instead, immediately devote 20 minutes to something relaxing. Play on the floor with the kids, spend some time stretching, take a warm shower, pick weeds in your garden or flowers for the dinner table. Suddenly you're not so starving, are you?

Don't eat alone.

People who sit down for at least one meal a day with family are more likely to be thinner, eat healthier, and have lower risks of major diseases. Just don't get so lost in conversation that you forget to savor each bite and in turn eat too quickly before realizing you are full (see "Keep your focus," on page 111).

Click before you eat.

University of Wisconsin-Madison researchers had 43 people take a snapshot of what they were going to eat before they ate it, and that simple act had a very sobering effect on their indulgences. One of the study subjects said, "Who wants to take a picture of a jumbo bag of M&Ms?" Finally ... a good use of your cell phone camera.

Eat only at the table.

There's a whole body of research that suggests that when you eat on the couch, at your desk, in the car, or standing at the sink, your brain doesn't always register the fact that you had a meal, and that can lead to feelings of deprivation and overeating later in the day. Even when you're just having a snack, take the time to put it on a plate (never eat right out of the bag or box), and then have a seat at the table with a glass of water or seltzer to enjoy with your mini-meal.

State your intentions.

You're sad or lonely or bored, and you're about to dive into a large bowl of ice cream. Okay, fine. But first admit what you're doing by saying out loud, "I'm not hungry, but I'm going to eat this anyway." Dr. Wansink of Cornell University asked volunteers to try this method, with great success. Simply taking time to think about what you're about to do may be enough to dissuade you from doing it.

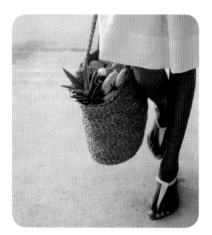

a tub of ice cream, buy individual bars or Popsicles. In fact, many foods now come in 100-calorie snack-pack portions. The less quantity that's available, the less you'll eat. (If you do have some degree of self-control, buy the larger package, read how many servings it contains, and put only 100 calories' worth on a plate for your snack—no going back for more!)

Reorganize your kitchen. Think of it this way: If you walk by a shoe store on your way home from work every day, eventually you're going to end up with a closet full of pumps. Likewise, if you pass a clear jar of oatmeal cookies on your counter every morning or see the leftover lo mein front and center when you open the fridge, you're going to be more inclined to indulge. So put that cookie jar on the top shelf of the pantry, replace the candy dish with a bowl of fruit, and put the carrot sticks, snap peas, and yogurt at eye level in the icebox.

STEP **4**

Devise an emergency distraction plan.

Back in the 1960s a psychology professor at Columbia University named Walter Mischel conducted a series of experiments that are still pertinent today. He put marshmallows or cookies in front of several four-year-olds. Before leaving the room, he told them they could either indulge immediately or wait to be rewarded with two treats when he returned. After doing this with hundreds of kids, he identified "distraction" as one successful strategy in avoiding temptation. In other words, the patient kids sang, counted, twirled their hair, or did something to take their minds off that marshmallow. It's easy for you to do this, too. Here are some ideas:

Get busy. Sometimes we end up nibbling just because we're bored. Keep idle hands and minds occupied by doing some needlework, clipping coupons, checking e-mail, listening to music, or doing that same marshmallow experiment with your kids. The more engrossed you become in something, the less you'll think about eating.

6 WAYS TO TELL IF YOU'RE REALLY HUNGRY

Your appetite signal can't be trusted. For proof, just look at all the overweight people in this country, who consume more calories than their bodies need. The next time you get the urge to eat, here's how to tell if your hunger is genuine.

1. Look for a slow build. Physical hunger comes on gradually, while emotional hunger is sudden.

2. Listen for the growl. When your stomach is truly empty, it'll feel hollow and you'll experience gurgling and hunger pangs.

3. Ask yourself what you're hungry for. True hunger can be satisfied with any food. If only a particular food will do, you're not really hungry.

4. Wait 10 minutes. Hit the timer on the stove or the one on your sports watch and distract yourself with a task until you hear the ding. Usually by that time, if it's a craving, it will have passed.

5. Drink 8 ounces of water. Many people confuse hunger with thirst, thinking they need food when their bodies actually need fluids. So drink a glass of water, then wait 10 minutes. If you're still hungry, it's legitimate.

6. Stick something else in your mouth. If gum, a lollipop, or a mint satisfies you, it's an oral craving, not hunger.

EXTREME EATERS

Over the last several decades, food manufacturers discovered that we all have a seemingly insatiable desire for sugar and salt, and they've responded by stuffing our food with mind-boggling amounts of these substances. We live in a world where a jar of tomato sauce can have more sugar per serving than vanilla ice cream. It's possible to get more salt from breakfast cereals than we do from French fries. This full-scale assault on our taste buds has the dangerous side effect of making us want more and more food. That's because processed foods place us on a flavor seesaw: We eat something terrifically sweet, and almost immediately we want to counter it with something salty. After which, it occurs to us that something with a little sugar would hit the spot nicely.

Manufacturers load foods with both salt and sugar for another reason: When salt and sugar hit critical levels in the same food, the combination trips satisfaction sensors in our brain similar to the ones activated in drug addicts when they get a fix. It's the manufacturer's way of making us addicted to their products.

The solution? Retrain your overwhelmed taste buds to remind them how to taste—and enjoy—subtler flavors again.

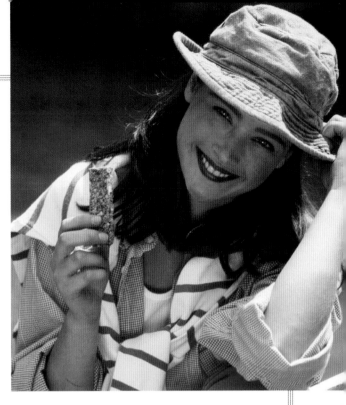

Add your own salt and sugar.

Buy unsweetened and low-salt versions of your favorite foods, then sprinkle on what you think is missing, gradually reducing the amount you add each time. The advantage to putting the seasoning on the surface of the food is that it will hit your tongue first, thereby reassuring you (and your brain) that you're getting the flavor you want.

Enjoy just a taste.

Regulate sugar intake by enjoying it in more moderate doses. Instead of eating a whole chocolate bar, enjoy an individually wrapped single-serving square. Instead of eating a modern-size brownie (today's brownie recipes serve 8, whereas the same recipe from 1936 served 12), cut a smaller piece and slowly savor every bite.

Check the first three ingredients.

If one of them is sugar or some other form of sweetener (white grape juice, dehydrated cane juice, honey, anything that has "syrup" in its name or ends in "-ose," such as dextrose or fructose), chances are you're holding an extremely sweet product. Unless it's a form of dessert, you'll want to pass on it. This is especially true for things that shouldn't be sweet to start with: Salad dressing, tomato sauce, soup, and

peanut butter. Healthy products like yogurt, instant oatmeal, and smoothies can contain loads of sugar as well.

Satisfy salt cravings with nuts.

Because of their fat and protein, nuts help keep you feeling full until your next meal. And that fat is "good" fat, the kind that's friendly to your heart. Shelling pistachios, peanuts, or sunflower seeds spreads out the amount of time it takes to eat your treat. That gives your brain time to register the calories you're taking in, and your snack will feel more satisfying.

Substitute less extreme snacks.

A bowl of juicy berries is just as likely to satisfy your sweet cravings as candy. Need a salt fix? Try celery with peanut butter; you can even make a few stalks in the morning before work and take them with you. The less extreme the flavors, the less likely you'll be sent chasing the opposite sensation.

Wean yourself from fast food.

If you typically eat a fast-food lunch with soda, start by having the meal with water. Even if you drink diet soda, go ahead and switch to water or seltzer because the dramatic sweetness of diet beverages still flips the craving switches in your brain and can cause you to overeat. Once you've adjusted to water, substitute salad for fries. Soon fast food will lose its allure.

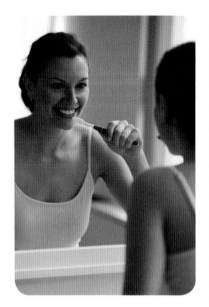

Daydream. Picture yourself in a peaceful setting—lying in a hammock under two beachside palm trees or in some other pleasant, natural, outdoor place you've visited. Use all your senses to recreate the experience until you feel like you're really there.

Take a sniff. Researchers discovered that when people sniff banana, green apple, or peppermint, they're better able to control their food cravings. See if it works for you by keeping those things in your kitchen or carrying a cotton ball soaked in an essential oil in a zip-close bag in your car or purse. (If the craving is really bad, take a whiff of your guy's workout shirt. That'll kill anybody's appetite.)

Brush your teeth. You wouldn't want to ruin that fresh, minty taste with some fatty snack, would you?

Pop an Altoid. These mints are so strong they'll change the taste of anything you eat for many minutes afterward. So if you're due at a meeting where there will be doughnuts or cookies on the table, pop one ahead of time. Fresh breath is the bonus.

THE TASTE OF TOOTHPASTE IN YOUR MOUTH IS A GREAT CRAVING-CRUSHER. BRUSH YOUR TEETH IMMEDIATELY AFTER EVERY MEAL TO SQUASH THE TEMPTATION FOR SECONDS.

Hold your nose. Ever notice how you tend to eat less during allergy season or when you have a cold? That's because a large percentage of our sense of taste is linked to our sense of smell. If you succumb to a craving, try pinching your nose closed or even plugging your nostrils with tissue while you eat. You'll be amazed at how bland the food tastes and how much less of it you'll want.

Think of your family or even your pet. Sometimes diverting your thoughts momentarily to those who love you, who matter more, or who bring you pleasure helps you instantly put things in perspective during very stressful moments.

STEP 5

Complete your reprogramming.

There's one other temptation-busting strategy that we can steal from those four-year-olds. When Dr. Mischel performed his marshmallow experiment (see step 4, page 116), he told the kids to imagine that those marshmallows were cotton balls or clouds, dramatically improving their ability to be patient and not partake. The marshmallow went from being an object of desire to merely an object, which made a big difference. So try doing a little rewiring in your head. Think of that piece of pizza you're craving as a triangular slice of the cardboard box it came in. Or imagine those chicken wings you're preparing to snarf down as being, well, real chicken wings. Taking the personality or emotion out of the food instantly makes it more resistible. Even envisioning it in black and white rather than color can work.

Another trick: Remove some of the pleasure you associate with consuming a food by changing where you eat it. Instead of munching popcorn from a big bowl while lounging on the living-room couch in front of the TV, pour a small amount onto a plate and force yourself to eat it at the kitchen table. Not the same, is it? Once you've altered the eating experience, you may find you've also changed how much you want the food.

If you're an emotional eater, all of these tools should help you cut hundreds of calories from your day and see real progress on the scale. Bonus: After you buy your Halloween candy this year (choose a kind you don't love), you'll have plenty left to put in trick-or-treaters' bags, where it belongs.

Sugar-Proof Your Diet

It's hiding in places you least expect it. Here's how to cut needless calories by being a smarter sugar sleuth.

Back in the days when humans carried clubs and dinner was a hit-or-miss proposition, our ancestors sought out fruits and other sweet foods for their taste and their calories. (Also, sweet foods were less likely to be poisonous than bitter foods.) They weren't worried about fitting into a size 0 bearskin; they just wanted to survive.

Today that natural sweet tooth remains, but it no longer works in our favor. There's simply too much sugar within easy reach. And today's sweetened foods are processed and highly concentrated. Unlike berries and whole fruits, they contain little protein, fat, or fiber to slow the absorption of sugar into the bloodstream. "The sugar gives you a fast source of energy, but it is quickly used up, leaving you hungry for more," says Lona Sandon, RD, assistant professor at the University of Texas Southwestern in Dallas and a spokesperson for the American Dietetic Association.

To keep us hooked on their products, manufacturers now add sugar to just about everything—even stuff like pretzels. Other surprising sources of sugar include fat-free products (to enhance taste), flavored foods (such as yogurt and oatmeal), and dressings and marinades. Even "natural" sources of sugar can still blow your calorie budget when condensed into a small serving. One 8-ounce glass of OJ, for instance, has the same amount of sugar as two whole oranges, says Sandon.

ARE YOU ADDICTED TO SUGAR?

The foods you crave the most are often the ones your body needs the least. And the more you eat them, the more you want them, especially when it comes to noshes high in simple carbohydrates and sugar. Switching to artificial sweeteners won't help; you'll still crave sweetness.

What will help? Going cold turkey. Swear off all sugary foods and drinks for two weeks and—*voilà*—your cravings will be gone, or at least diminished to the point where you can safely ignore them.

You know the obvious foods to avoid: cookies, candy bars, ice cream, pancakes with maple syrup, and the like. But also pay attention to these land mines:

- Soft drinks (diet or regular): These are the biggest source of sugar in today's diet.
- Fruit drinks and fruit juice: Even if it's 100 percent fruit juice, it's largely sugar. Stick to 6 ounces a day.
- Breakfast cereal: Starting off the day with sugar sets you up for sugar cravings later on. Look for cereals with no more than 8 grams of sugar per serving.
- Packaged foods: Manufacturers find ways to put sugar in just about everything to keep you hooked on their products, from peanut butter to baked beans. Aim to limit all added sugars to no more than 10 teaspoons (40 grams) a day.

The American Heart Association recommends that women limit added sugar to 100 calories (6 teaspoons, or 25 grams) and men to 150 calories (9 teaspoons, or 37 grams) per day. Most of us consume more than three times that amount. To cut back, read the Nutrition Facts label and the ingredient list on packaged foods. Look at the grams of sugar, opting for products that include less for the same portion. To find hidden sugar on the ingredients list, look for words ending in "-ose" (dextrose, maltose, glucose)

TASTY LOW-SUGAR ALTERNATIVES

	HIGH-SUGAR SURPRISE	LOW-SUGAR SWAP
1	**Newman's Own marinara sauce** 11 g sugar, 70 cal per ½ cup	**Muir Glen Organic tomato basil pasta sauce** 4 g sugar, 60 cal per ½ cup
2	**Breyers Fruit on the Bottom strawberry yogurt** 28 g sugar, 170 cal per 6 ounces	**Fage 2% strawberry-flavored Greek yogurt** 17 g sugar, 130 cal per 5.3 ounces
3	**Edensoy vanilla soymilk** 16 g sugar, 150 cal per 8 ounces	**Silk vanilla soymilk** 7 g sugar, 100 cal per 8 ounces
4	**Honey Nut Cheerios Milk 'n' Cereal Bar** 14 g sugar, 160 cal	**Nature Valley Oats 'n' Honey granola bar** 6 g sugar, 90 cal
5	**Skippy Natural peanut butter** 3 g sugar, 180 cal per 2 tablespoons	**Arrowhead Mills peanut butter** 1 g sugar, 190 cal per 2 tablespoons

as well as additives such as cane sugar, syrup, honey, corn syrup, high-fructose corn syrup, cane juice, and dextrin. Ingredients appear in descending order of weight, so if one or more code words appear in the first three or four positions, the food probably contains lots of sugar.

Compare the familiar products below, which are surprisingly high in sugar, with some equally tasty lower-in-sugar alternatives.

	HIGH-SUGAR SURPRISE	LOW-SUGAR SWAP
6	**Heinz vegetarian beans** 14 g sugar, 140 cal per ½ cup	**Amy's Organic vegetarian beans** 9 g sugar, 120 cal per ½ cup
7	**Ken's Italian salad dressing** 4 g sugar, 90 cal per 2 tablespoons	**Kraft Viva Italian salad dressing** 1 g sugar, 90 cal per 2 tablespoons
8	**Dole pineapple chunks in heavy syrup** 22 g sugar, 90 cal per ½ cup	**Del Monte crushed pineapple in 100% juice** 14 g sugar, 60 cal per ½ cup
9	**Quaker instant oatmeal, maple and brown sugar flavor** 13 g sugar, 160 cal per packet	**Erewhon organic instant oatmeal, maple spice flavor** 4 g sugar, 130 cal per packet
10	**Minute Maid orange juice** 24 g sugar, 110 cal per 8 ounces	**Tropicana 50 orange juice** 10 g of sugar, 50 cal per 8 ounces
11	**Ken's Teriyaki marinade** 3 g sugar, 20 cal per tablespoon	**Mrs. Dash mesquite grille marinade** 1 g sugar, 25 cal per tablespoon

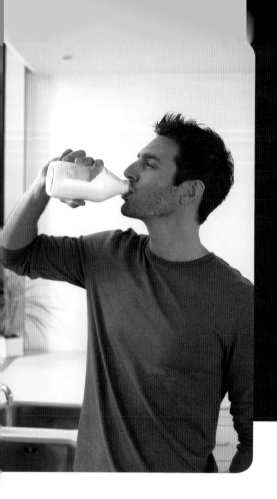

Top 20
Power Foods for Walkers

You're walking to lose weight. Great! Now make sure your diet is helping, not hurting, your efforts. If you're filling up on low-fat snacks to curb hunger, relying on fast-digesting carbohydrates for fuel, or eating protein-poor salads to cut calories, we have far better suggestions.

Your food should do three things for your body: provide lasting energy, keep your blood sugar levels steady, and of course, fill you up. Lean protein, "good" fats, and slow-digesting complex carbs are the nutrients that get the job done, and you'll get plenty of each from the following 12 power foods.

Meals rich in these foods not only keep you satisfied, they increase levels of leptin, a hormone that reins in hunger and decreases levels of ghrelin, a hormone that bumps up hunger. They also limit the rise in blood sugar after a meal. That's important: People whose diets boost blood sugar the most tend to have more body fat, especially around the abdomen. A diet that causes your blood sugar to spike and dive may even slow your metabolism.

Look to these 20 foods and beverages to power up your diet, and you'll have the energy to make it up that hill, the satisfied feeling to help ward off snack attacks, and the body chemistry that will begin melting the pounds away.

1 Low-Fat Milk

If you left milk behind in your childhood, you may be missing out. Two Harvard studies found that people who made dairy foods part of their daily diets were 21 percent less likely to develop insulin resistance, a condition that makes it harder for your body to use glucose and easier for it to store foods as fat. Milk is rich in calcium and vitamin D, good for bones. And low-fat dairy is a cornerstone of the DASH diet, shown to lower blood pressure. Choose low-fat or skim milk instead of 2 percent.

2 Low-Fat Yogurt

It's hard to find a snack that's rich in protein yet low in fat, but low-fat yogurt is one of them. It's also a great source of bone-building calcium, and the live beneficial bacteria help keep your gut happy and your immune system going strong. It's a great base for smoothies, and it's a lower-fat substitute for some or all of the mayonnaise in creamy salads and the sour cream in baked goods, soups, and chip dips. Choose low-fat yogurt that's not overly sweetened, and look for "live active cultures" on the container.

YOGURT IS A GREAT SOURCE OF BONE-BUILDING CALCIUM.

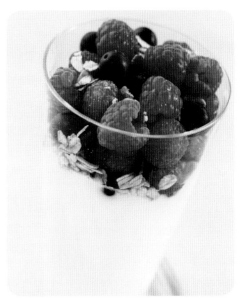

3 Swiss Cheese

A review of more than 90 studies in the journal *Nutrition Reviews* revealed a strong link between high-calcium intake and improved body composition. "If you don't have adequate calcium in your diet, any attempt at weight loss will be less productive," says Robert P. Heaney, MD, a professor at Creighton University in Omaha, Nebraska, and lead study author.

When your calcium intake is low, your body secretes hormones that allow you to make better use of the calcium in your diet. Problem is, at the same time, your body signals fat cells to hold on to fat. Dairy, especially Swiss cheese, along with low-fat milk and yogurt, are the preferred sources of calcium. Eat three servings of dairy a day.

4 Green Tea

You'll not only fight winter's chill by sipping green tea, you'll also shrink your belly, especially if you're walking, too, according to a study in the *Journal of Nutrition*. Study participants drank a beverage containing catechins—powerful antioxidant compounds in green tea—or a beverage with no catechins. They also did about 180 minutes of moderate-intensity exercise, mainly walking, each week. After 12 weeks green-tea drinkers lost 7.4 percent more abdominal fat than non–green tea drinkers.

"Catechins increase metabolism and the rate at which the liver burns fat," says study author Kevin C. Maki, PhD. To reap those rewards, drink four to six cups of caffeinated green tea a day and log at least 180 minutes of exercise each week.

5 Oats

OATS ARE ONE OF THE BEST SOURCES OF PLANT-BASED PROTEIN.

Many cereals lack significant fiber or digest too quickly, leaving you hungry again before lunch. A better bet is oatmeal. Oats are one of the best sources of plant-based protein, and their soluble fiber forms a gel in the stomach that slows digestion, critical for heading off blood sugar spikes and keeping hunger under control. Oatmeal is known to lower cholesterol, and it's estimated that eating it five or six times a week can reduce the risk of type 2 diabetes by as much as 39 percent. Note that steel-cut oats are the least processed, but even instant oats are a good source of fiber.

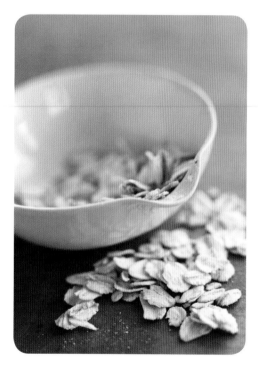

6 Barley

Enjoy a delicious barley side dish instead of white rice with dinner and you could be well on your way to shedding dangerous belly fat, according to a report in the *American Journal of Clinical Nutrition*. In the study, people on a reduced-calorie diet either were told to avoid whole-grain foods or to get all their grain servings from whole grains (such as whole wheat bread, oatmeal, barley, and brown rice) for 12 weeks. A grain product fit the bill if a whole grain was the first ingredient on the nutrition label. Although both groups lost equal amounts of weight, the whole-grain group lost more abdominal fat.

A good rule of thumb: Make sure you get at least three servings of whole-grain foods a day. (A serving is a slice of bread, an ounce of cold cereal, or a half cup of cooked cereal, rice, pasta, or other grain.) Oatmeal and barley are particularly good choices because they're rich in soluble fiber and don't typically raise blood sugar as much as white or brown rice.

7 Beans

Not only are they incredibly filling, they also pack a heap of nutrition in a relatively low-calorie package. Better still, some of the starch in beans is a type called resistant starch, which the body can't even digest, so the calories don't count. Beans also have a secret ingredient: soluble fiber. It not only lowers cholesterol but steadies blood-sugar levels for lasting energy.

For an added bonus, it turns out that beans really are good for your heart! And a recent study by the U.S. Department of Agriculture ranked beans among the top 10 foods richest in antioxidants. Try canned or dried beans, from black, red, and white, to everything in between, like cranberry, Roman, or garbanzo.

8 Quinoa

Quinoa is a high-protein grain that provides all nine of the essential amino acids, making it what's known as a "complete protein." It's also loaded with lysine, which is essential for tissue growth and repair, as well as magnesium, iron, copper, and phosphorus. It's a light and tasty alternative to rice as a side dish and works nicely in soups and salads, too. And it has no gluten!

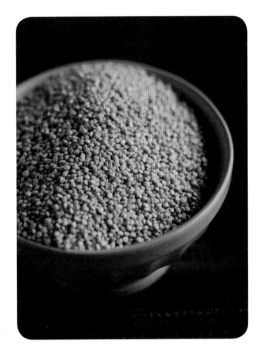

9 Eggs

Protein helps with weight loss in a number of ways. First, your body uses more energy (think calories) to break down protein foods than it does to break down other foods. Protein also helps you hang on to muscle mass as you're losing weight, and since muscle burns more calories than fat, you want to keep as much of it as you can. Finally, protein dampens hunger better than carbs do.

QUINOA IS A HIGH-PROTEIN GRAIN THAT PROVIDES ALL NINE OF THE ESSENTIAL AMINO ACIDS.

Include a source of protein at every meal, especially breakfast, where most people fall short. Eggs are an easy and inexpensive solution. A hard-boiled egg even makes a great snack, especially when you might otherwise reach for some chips or a candy bar. Eggs are also one of nature's few good food sources of vitamin D, which preliminary research suggests could play an important role in keeping weight off.

10 Walnuts

Studies point to nuts as a waist-friendly addition to your diet, as long as you don't go overboard. Chalk it up to their fiber, their protein, and their "good" fat, which may increase the body's sensitivity to insulin, aiding weight loss. Walnuts are one of the best non-fish sources of omega-3 fats, which is excellent for warding off heart disease and can help prevent type 2 diabetes. They're also rich in vitamin E, an important antioxidant that may help fight prostate and lung cancers.

11 Almonds

Making your diet a little nuttier could help shrink your belly. According to a study from the Archives of Internal Medicine, more than 1,200 adults were put into one of three diet groups. One followed a Mediterranean diet and ate an ounce of nuts daily, a second followed a Mediterranean diet while consuming a liter of olive oil every week, and a third served as a control. Only the group eating nuts decreased their abdominal fat. Like peanuts and walnuts, almonds contain plant sterols, which have been shown to lower cholesterol. Almonds also provide an extra benefit in the form of bone-building calcium.

12 Salmon

Eating fat might sound like a crazy idea, but getting more omega-3 fatty acids from fatty fish like salmon could be just what the diet doctor ordered, according to a study in the *British Journal of Nutrition.* "Although the exact mechanisms are unknown, omega-3 fatty acids reduce fat mass," says Irene Munro, study author and researcher from the University of Newcastle in Newcastle, Australia. Other studies have found that omega-3 fatty acids make you feel less hungry and more satisfied up to two hours after eating a fatty-fish meal. Aim to eat salmon or another oily fish, like mackerel, herring, or canned tuna, at least twice a week.

IF EATEN DAILY, BLUEBERRIES CAN HELP KEEP YOUR EYES HEALTHY, BRAIN AND MEMORY SHARP, AND REDUCE YOUR RISK OF HEART DISEASE AND CANCER.

13 Chicken

Chicken is a good source of the antioxidant mineral selenium as well as B vitamins. Eating chicken for protein will help ensure that you lose fat, not muscle. Bonus: Your body takes a while to break down protein, and this slows the digestion of the whole meal, including the carbs it contains, making for a slower rise in blood sugar. Best yet: Protein puts a damper on hunger, expanding the time between when you eat and when your stomach starts rumbling again.

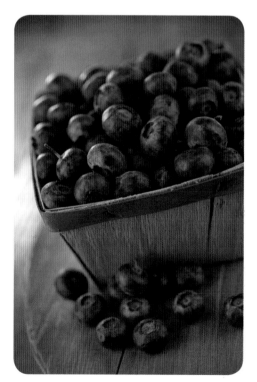

14 Blueberries

Blueberries are rich in powerful disease-fighting antioxidants. Studies show that if you make blueberries a daily indulgence, they can help keep your eyes healthy, reduce your risk of heart disease and cancer, and help to keep your brain and memory sharp. They're also full of fiber and natural plant compounds called anthocyanins, which can help keep your blood sugar in check.

15 Grapefruit

Citrus fruits, especially grapefruit, contain a flavonoid called naringenin. In a study in the journal *Diabetes,* some mice on a high-fat diet were given supplemental naringenin, and others weren't. In the end the naringenin almost completely prevented a gain in body fat. Whether the same results apply to humans and how much we'd need to eat is unclear at this point, although other studies have found that grapefruit can speed weight loss.

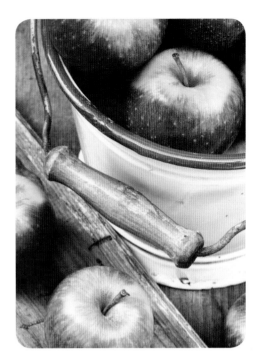

16 Apples

Can eating an apple a day really keep the doctor away? It certainly can help control blood sugar, which in turn helps prevent type 2 diabetes. Apples contain an impressive 4 g of fiber, which lowers cholesterol, as well antioxidant compounds called flavonoids, believed to reduce the risk of cancer and heart disease.

17 Pears

Like apples, pears contain flavonoids, which are natural chemicals in plant foods that aid in fat burning. They're also a great source of fiber, vitamin C, and vitamin E. And at only 100 calories a serving, you get a lot of sweet bang for the buck.

APPLES CONTAIN ANTIOXIDANT COMPOUNDS BELIEVED TO REDUCE THE RISK OF CANCER AND HEART DISEASE.

18 Bell Peppers

Sweet peppers are famously loaded with fiber, vitamin A, and vitamin C. And like apples and pears, they've got those awesome flavonoids, too. Women who consumed the most flavonoids had significantly lower increases in body mass index over a 14-year period than women who ate the least, according to a study in the American Journal of Clinical Nutrition. "Animal studies have shown that these flavonoids can increase energy [calorie] expenditure, increase glucose uptake into muscle, and increase fat burning," says Laura Hughes, MSc, the study's lead investigator and a nutritional epidemiologist at Maastricht University in the Netherlands. Onions, leeks, and green and white tea also contain flavonoids.

19 Flaxseed

These shiny, nutty-tasting seeds pack a secret weight-loss weapon: compounds called lignans. Consumption of lignans in postmenopausal women was associated with lower body fat and body mass index, according to a study in the *British Journal of Nutrition*. "Previous studies in mice show that lignans reduce adipose [fat] tissue mass," says Anne-Sophie Morisset, DtP, MSc, lead study author from Laval University in Quebec City, Canada, so it wasn't a huge surprise that eating lignans led to weight

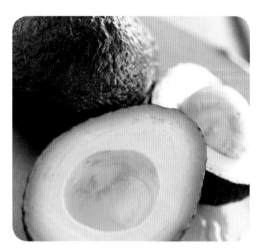

loss in women. Morisset recommends grinding and adding a tablespoon of flaxseed each day to cereals, yogurt, or salad dressing. Other sources of lignans include sesame seeds, multigrain bread, hummus, garlic, dried apricots, dates, soybeans, sunflower seeds, and pistachios.

20 Avocados

These creamy treats are loaded with monounsaturated fat, the same heart-healthy kind found in olive oil. Diets rich in this type of fat keep blood-sugar levels steady and may help you trim inches from your waistline if you keep your portion sizes in check. Avocados also contain more protein and cholesterol-lowering soluble fiber than any other fruit.

AVOCADOS CONTAIN MORE PROTEIN AND CHOLESTEROL-LOWERING SOLUBLE FIBER THAN ANY OTHER FRUIT.

Avocados are rich in sterols, the compounds that lower cholesterol. They're also packed with vitamins and minerals, including magnesium, vitamin C, folate, and zinc. Ounce for ounce they provide more potassium than bananas! Add some avocado to a sandwich or anything else with carbs, and the fat will slow digestion of the meal, thus making it easier on your blood sugar. Of course, even with "good" fat comes some calories, so you don't want to start eating avocados with total abandon. Luckily, a little avocado goes a long way.

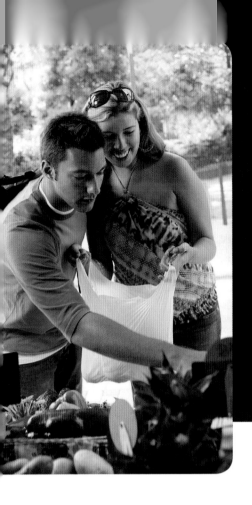

A Month of Walk It Off *Meals*

Take a month to change the way you eat. It's simple: Prepare the simple breakfast, lunch, and dinner recipes you'll see mapped out across one month on the meal calendar on the next page. Each day choose two items from the Snack Attack list on page 133, one for midmorning and one for midafternoon. All of the meal and snack choices feature foods or ingredients from our Top 20 Power Foods for Walkers list—all foods that boost energy and metabolism. Making better food choices every day will turbocharge your weight loss—and you'll feel like a million bucks, too!

Recipes for the dishes on the Walk It Off menus follow, with nutritional analyses for each. Several of the breakfast and lunch recipes freeze well, so they make great make-ahead meals that are good options when you're pinched for time. You can also enjoy leftover dinner dishes for lunch the next day or substitute a meal from another day to suit your tastes. That's all you need to start eating well to walk it off.

	Sunday	Monday	Tuesday
WEEK 1	**BREAKFAST** Yogurt Surprise **LUNCH** Cold Sesame Noodles and Vegetables **DINNER** Chicken with Apples and Calvados	**BREAKFAST** Oatmeal Blueberry Muffin **LUNCH** Cuban Bean Burrito **DINNER** Soy-Marinated Pork Tenderloin	**BREAKFAST** Classic One-Eye **LUNCH** Curried Chicken Salad Sandwich **DINNER** Cajun Shrimp and Crab Jambalaya
WEEK 2	**BREAKFAST** Greek Omelet **LUNCH** Feta Barley Salad with Citrus Dresing **DINNER** Fish Tacos	**BREAKFAST** Homemade Granola Bar **LUNCH** Turkey Swiss Wrap **DINNER** Asian Chicken Salad	**BREAKFAST** Yogurt Surprise **LUNCH** Quinoa and Chickpea Salad **DINNER** Green Pork Chili
WEEK 3	**BREAKFAST** Savory Oatmeal **LUNCH** Cuban Bean Burrito **DINNER** Baltimore Seafood Cakes	**BREAKFAST** Corn Waffles with Fresh Fruit Salsa **LUNCH** Broccoli and Cheese Calzone **DINNER** Asian BBQ Beef with Water Chestnut Salad	**BREAKFAST** Spicy Egg-and-Cheese Scramble **LUNCH** Feta Barley Salad with Citrus Dressing **DINNER** Grilled Jamaican Jerk Chicken
WEEK 4	**BREAKFAST** Baked Oatmeal Cup **LUNCH** Lettuces with Pears, Dates, and Manchego Cheese **DINNER** Sizzling Beef Fajitas	**BREAKFAST** Nutty Breakfast Smoothie **LUNCH** Sesame Chicken Wrap **DINNER** Lentil and Bean Chili	**BREAKFAST** Homemade Granola Bar **LUNCH** Barley, Black Bean, and Avocado Salad **DINNER** Santa Fe Stuffed Peppers

Wednesday	Thursday	Friday	Saturday
BREAKFAST Corn Waffles with Fresh Fruit Salsa **LUNCH** Pesto Tuna Wrap **DINNER** Asian BBQ Beef with Water Chestnut Salad	**BREAKFAST** Spicy Egg-and-Cheese Scramble **LUNCH** BLT Pasta Salad **DINNER** Grilled Jamaican Jerk Chicken	**BREAKFAST** Apple Bran Muffin **LUNCH** Lemony Lentil and Vegetable Salad **DINNER** Penne with Fresh Tomato Sauce and Grilled Zucchini	**BREAKFAST** Savory Oatmeal **LUNCH** Broccoli and Cheese Calzone **DINNER** Santa Fe Stuffed Peppers
BREAKFAST Baked Oatmeal Cup **LUNCH** Cold Sesame Noodles and Vegetables **DINNER** Caribbean Seafood Curry Stew	**BREAKFAST** Peanut Butter and Blueberry Mash on Whole Wheat Toast **LUNCH** Black Bean and Grapefruit Salad **DINNER** Southwestern Shepherd's Pie	**BREAKFAST** Oatmeal Blueberry Muffin **LUNCH** Sesame Chicken Wrap **DINNER** Lentil and Bean Chili	**BREAKFAST** Nutty Breakfast Smoothie **LUNCH** BLT Pasta Salad **DINNER** Chicken Kabobs with Cherry Tomatoes
BREAKFAST Apple Bran Muffin **LUNCH** Hummus and Pepper Jack Wrap **DINNER** Salmon As You Like It	**BREAKFAST** Yogurt Surprise **LUNCH** Curried Chicken Salad Sandwich **DINNER** Veggie Tacos with Homemade Salsa and Guacamole	**BREAKFAST** Peanut Butter and Blueberry Mash on Whole Wheat Toast **LUNCH** Pesto Tuna Wrap **DINNER** Soy-Marinated Pork Tenderloin	**BREAKFAST** Greek Omelet **LUNCH** Lemony Lentil and Vegetable Salad **DINNER** Chicken with Apple and Calvados
BREAKFAST Classic One-Eye **LUNCH** Cuban Bean Burrito **DINNER** Asian Chicken Salad	**BREAKFAST** Blueberry Oatmeal Muffin **LUNCH** Quinoa and Chickpea Salad **DINNER** Cajun Shrimp and Crab Jambalaya	**BREAKFAST** Corn Waffles with Fresh Fruit Salsa **LUNCH** Broccoli and Cheese Calzone **DINNER** Chicken Kabobs with Cherry Tomatoes	**BREAKFAST** Spicy Egg-and-Cheese Scramble **LUNCH** Cold Sesame Noodles and Vegetables **DINNER** Veggie Tacos with Homemade Salsa and Guacamole

Oatmeal Blueberry Muffins

The combination of grated orange zest and blueberries is refreshing all year round. Eat one and freeze the rest for a grab-and-go meal or fill muffin tins with batter the night before, refrigerate, and pop them in the oven first thing in the morning.

MAKES 12 • PREP TIME: 45 MINUTES

¾ cup plus 2 tablespoons whole wheat flour

¾ cup all-purpose flour

1½ teaspoons baking powder

½ teaspoon baking soda

¼ teaspoon salt

1 teaspoon ground cinnamon

1 cup plus 2 tablespoons old-fashioned rolled oats

1 large egg

2 large egg whites

½ cup maple syrup

¾ cup low-fat buttermilk

3 tablespoons canola oil

2 teaspoons grated orange zest

1 tablespoon orange juice

1 teaspoon vanilla extract

1½ cups fresh blueberries, rinsed and patted dry

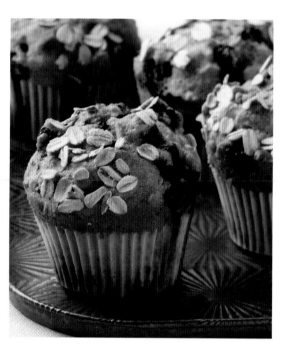

1 Preheat oven to 400°F (204°C). Lightly coat with cooking spray a muffin pan that holds 12 standard-size muffin cups or insert paper liners.

2 In a large bowl, whisk together whole wheat flour, all-purpose flour, baking powder, baking soda, salt, and cinnamon. Stir in 1 cup rolled oats.

3 In a medium bowl, whisk egg, egg whites, and syrup until smooth. Add buttermilk, oil, orange zest, orange juice, and vanilla and whisk until blended. Add to the flour mixture and mix with a rubber spatula just until dry ingredients are moistened. Fold in blueberries. Spoon batter into muffin cups, filling them almost to the top. Sprinkle tops with remaining 2 tablespoons rolled oats.

4 Bake until muffins are lightly browned and tops spring back when touched, 18 to 22 minutes. Loosen the edges of the muffins, turn out onto a wire rack, and let cool slightly before serving. One serving is 1 muffin.

Per serving: 180 calories, 5 g total fat, (0 g saturated), 30 g carbohydrates, 5 g protein, 3 g fiber, 18 mg cholesterol, 190 mg sodium

Nutty Breakfast Smoothie

The almond butter gives this smoothie a nice nutty twist. Experiment by substituting apple juice or skim milk for the orange juice.

MAKES 1 • PREP TIME: 5 minutes

½ cup plain nonfat yogurt

1 banana

1 tablespoon almond butter

½ teaspoon flaxseed

¾ cup orange juice (natural, not from concentrate)

Dash of cinnamon

Puree in a blender or food processor until smooth.

Per serving: 348 calories, 11 g fat (1 g saturated), 60 g carbohydrates, 10 g protein, 4 g fiber, 3 mg cholesterol, 71 mg sodium

SNACK ATTACK

Snacking isn't evil; it's what you snack on that's the problem. In fact, snacking is an effective way to control and even lose weight because it prevents you from becoming ravenously hungry and overeating at mealtime. But smart snacking requires advance planning. Keep these 10 "safe snacks" on hand for mid-morning or mid-afternoon pick-me-ups that will stabilize blood sugar, stave off cravings until mealtime, and keep your metabolism humming all day.

- Handful of unsalted mixed nuts (almonds, walnuts, pecans) and dried cranberries
- Hard-boiled egg
- 4 cups of air-popped popcorn
- Cup of low-fat yogurt, ½ sliced Granny Smith apple for dipping
- 20 red seedless grapes (try them frozen!)
- Stick of low-fat string cheese
- Frozen fruit bar
- 1 celery stick with one tablespoon of peanut butter
- Apple
- Cup of snack-size raw veggies (carrots, peppers, cherry tomatoes)

Greek Omelet

Top this Mediterranean dish with a ½ tablespoon of chopped black olives, diced red onion, or capers to add an extra tang to your morning.

Makes 1 • PREP TIME: 15 minutes

2 large eggs

¼ cup cooked chopped spinach, squeezed to remove water

¼ cup crumbled feta cheese (about 2 ounces)

¼ to ½ teaspoon dried oregano, to taste

Coarse salt and pepper

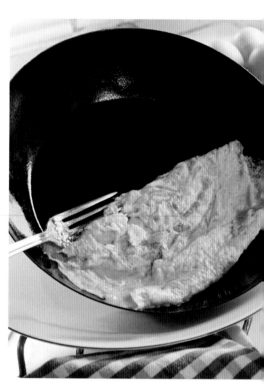

1 Spray a skillet with cooking spray and place over medium heat. Beat eggs and pour into skillet. Cook for a minute, shaking pan to evenly distribute eggs.

2 Sprinkle spinach and feta cheese over eggs, then top with oregano, salt, and pepper. When eggs are nearly set, fold omelet in half with a spatula and cook a minute more to finish.

Per serving: 225 calories, 15 g fat (6 g saturated), 4 g carbohydrates, 438 mg cholesterol, 19 g protein, 2 g fiber, 442 mg sodium

Apple Bran Muffins

The wheat bran in this recipe provides a healthy dose of fiber, while the applesauce keeps these muffins super moist for days.

Makes 12 • PREP TIME: 30 minutes

2 large eggs

½ cup packed light brown sugar

1 cup unsweetened applesauce

¾ cup low-fat buttermilk

1 cup unprocessed wheat bran

3 tablespoons canola oil

1 teaspoon vanilla extract

1 cup whole wheat flour

¾ cup all-purpose flour

1½ teaspoons baking powder

½ teaspoon baking soda

¼ teaspoon salt

2 teaspoons ground cinnamon

¼ teaspoon ground nutmeg

1 cup chopped peeled apple (1 medium)

⅓ cup chopped walnuts

1 Preheat oven to 400°F (204°C). Lightly coat with cooking spray a muffin pan that holds 12 standard-size muffin cups or insert paper liners.

2 In a medium bowl, whisk eggs and brown sugar until smooth. Add applesauce, buttermilk, wheat bran, oil, and vanilla and whisk until blended.

3 In a large bowl, whisk together whole wheat flour, all-purpose flour, baking powder, baking soda, salt, cinnamon, and nutmeg. Add the egg mixture and mix with a rubber spatula just until the dry ingredients are moistened. Fold in apple. Spoon batter into muffin cups and sprinkle with walnuts.

4 Bake until tops of muffins are golden brown and spring back when touched lightly, 18 to 22 minutes. Let cool in pan for 5 minutes, then loosen the edges of the muffins and turn out onto a wire rack. Let cool slightly before serving.

Per serving: 194 calories, 7 g total fat (1 g saturated), 31 g carbohydrates, 5 g protein, 4 g fiber, 36 mg cholesterol, 194 mg sodium

Baked Oatmeal Cups

Although baked in a muffin tin, this delicious breakfast treat is eaten with a fork. Top with different berries or nuts to create a new taste each time.

Makes 12 • PREP TIME: 15 minutes (plus 45 minutes for baking)

3 cups rolled oats

3 cups quick-cooking oats

½ cup chopped and lightly toasted walnut pieces

1 tablespoon plus 1 teaspoon baking powder

1 teaspoon salt

1 cup canola oil

1 cup sugar

¼ cup brown sugar

1 ½ teaspoons cinnamon

4 eggs

2½ cups milk

Raisins, blueberries, bananas or any other fruit in season, for topping

1 Preheat oven to 350°F (177°C). Lightly coat with cooking spray a muffin pan that holds 12 standard-size muffin cups.

2 In a large bowl, combine oats, walnuts, baking powder, and salt. In another bowl, whisk together oil, sugar, brown sugar, cinnamon, and eggs.

3 Add oat mixture to egg mixture and stir to combine. Add milk; then distribute evenly in muffin cups.

4 Bake for 40 to 45 minutes, or until tops are golden brown and spring back lightly when touched.

5 Let cool slightly; then serve a baked oatmeal cup in a bowl, topped with raisins or fresh fruit and, if you like, a splash of milk over the top.

Per serving: (without fruit topping) 477 calories, 27 g fat (3 g saturated), 52 g carbohydrates, 10 g protein, 4 g fiber, 74 mg cholesterol, 382 mg sodium

Peanut Butter and Blueberry Mash on Whole Wheat Toast

Blueberries are an excellent source of fiber, and they are packed with vitamin C. Combined with peanut butter, this meal gives you staying power. Serve with a nice cold glass of low-fat milk to make this an almost perfect quick breakfast.

Serves 1 • PREP TIME: 5 minutes

1 slice whole wheat bread

2 tablespoons smooth or crunchy peanut butter, preferably natural

¼ cup blueberries, gently smashed with the back of a spoon

Toast bread, spread with peanut butter, and top with blueberry mash. That's it!

Per serving: 280 calories, 17 g fat (4 g saturated), 23 g carbohydrates, 12 g protein, 5 g fiber, 0 mg cholesterol, 282 mg sodium

SAVORY OATMEAL....ANY TIME OF DAY

Oatmeal isn't just for breakfast anymore. It all depends on what you choose to add to this hearty, healthy grain. From diced ham and cheese to bacon and sautéed leeks, the choice of tasty add-ins are endless. Below are just a few of the flavorful combinations worth trying:

- A swirl of top-quality olive oil, sea salt, cracked pepper, and a hint of fresh grated Parmesan cheese
- Diced ham and shredded cheddar cheese
- Sauteed chanterelle or shiitake mushrooms and grated Gruyére cheese
- Diced crispy-cooked pancetta or bacon and sautéed leeks
- A swirl of top-quality olive oil, diced tomato, avocado, and green onion
- Crumbled cooked sausage and sautéed peppers and onions
- A slight swirl of soy sauce and thinly sliced green onions, topped with a poached or soft-boiled egg
- Chopped walnuts, sliced grapes, and gorgonzola cheese

NOTE: Prepare your favorite instant or slow-cook oatmeal as directed. If you prefer your oatmeal on the moist side, instead of using milk, use a hint of olive oil, chicken broth, or butter.

Corn Waffles with Fresh Fruit Salsa

The cornmeal in this recipe makes these crisp, golden waffles taste so much like cornbread you could even top them with chicken and apples for a fabulous dinner.

Makes 12 to 14 • PREP TIME: 30 minutes

For the salsa:
½ cup mixed berries (blueberries, blackberries, or diced strawberries)

½ cup diced banana, kiwi, peach, or papaya

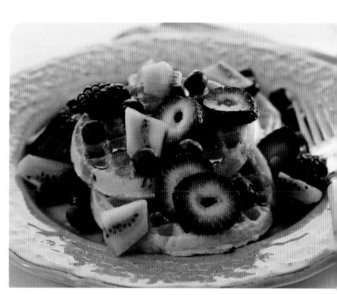

TIP Grind flaxseed to a coarse meal using an electric spice mill, a clean coffee grinder, or a blender. Flaxseeds need to be ground in order for your body to reap the full nutritional benefits.

For the waffles:
1½ cups cornmeal

½ cup whole wheat flour

½ cup all-purpose flour

2 tablespoons flaxseed

1 tablespoon baking powder

1 teaspoon salt

3 tablespoons sugar

2½ cups low-fat buttermilk

¼ cup canola oil

1 Preheat a waffle iron.

2 To make the salsa, in a small bowl, mix together fruit and set aside.

3 Meanwhile, in a large bowl, mix cornmeal, whole wheat flour, all-purpose flour, flaxseed, baking powder, salt, and sugar. Whisk in buttermilk and oil until batter is smooth.

4 Lightly coat heated waffle iron with cooking spray, then add 2/3 cup batter and cook until crisp and golden brown at the edges, about 5 minutes.

Serve immediately, topped with a spoonful of fruit salsa.

Per serving: (1 waffle with fruit topping) 190 calories, 6 g fat (1 g saturated), 29 g carbohydrates, 5 g protein, 3 g fiber, 2 mg cholesterol, 352 mg sodium

Homemade Granola Bars

Swap out the raisins or cranberries for carob chips to create a more sinful version of this nifty breakfast or snack bar.

Makes 16 • PREP TIME: 30 minutes (plus 1 hour to chill)

2 tablespoons unsalted butter, plus a bit for the baking dish

¾ cup honey or agave syrup

3 cups old-fashioned rolled oats

1½ cups slivered almonds (about 6 ounces)

Pinch coarse salt

1 cup raisins or dried cranberries

⅓ cup creamy peanut or almond butter

¼ cup light brown sugar

1 Preheat oven to 325°F (163°C).

2 In a small saucepan over low heat, melt butter and ¼ cup of either honey or agave syrup.

3 In a large bowl, mix together oats, almonds, and salt. Add butter mixture and stir to combine.

4 On a high-rimmed cookie sheet, distribute oat mixture evenly. Bake until golden, about 20 minutes, stirring twice while baking.

5 Remove oat mixture from oven and let cool completely on a wire rack. Return mixture to large bowl and mix in raisins or cranberries to combine well.

6 Butter an 8-inch (20-cm) baking dish. In your small saucepan, combine ½ cup honey or agave syrup, peanut or almond butter, and brown sugar and bring to a boil over medium heat. When sugar has completely dissolved, drizzle over oat mixture and mix well.

7 Transfer oat mixture to baking dish, pressing firmly with a rubber spatula. Refrigerate until firm, about 1 hour. Cut into 16 portions and store in an airtight container or freeze for future use.

Per serving: 247 calories, 10 g fat (2 g saturated), 37 g carbohydrates, 6 g protein, 3 g fiber, 4 mg cholesterol, 29 mg sodium

Classic One-Eye

A tablespoon of green or red salsa on the side of this cowboy favorite is nice, as is a hint of grated Parmesan dusted over the top.

Serves 1 • PREP TIME: 15 minutes

2 slices whole wheat bread

4 teaspoons unsalted butter

2 large eggs

Coarse salt and ground pepper

1 With a 2-inch (5-cm)-round cookie cutter or a small glass, cut a circle out of the center of both pieces of bread, reserving cutouts. Over medium-high heat, melt 2 teaspoons butter in a large nonstick skillet. When butter is foaming, add bread and cutouts and cook until toasted on the undersides.

2 Add 1 teaspoon butter to the hole in each piece of bread. Crack one egg into each hole and season with salt and pepper. Cook until egg whites are set (around a minute), then carefully flip the bread and cutouts and cook 2 minutes more.

3 Serve immediately, with cutouts on the side for dipping in the yolk.

Per serving: 208 calories, 13 g fat (7 g saturated), 12 g carbohydrates, 10 g protein, 2 g fiber, 232 mg cholesterol, 203 mg sodium

Yogurt Surprise

Made in a tall glass, this yogurt parfait is a deliciously healthy way to start your day. It's basically dessert for breakfast! And with the extra boost of protein Greek yogurt provides, you'll end up feeling satisfied for hours.

Makes 1 • prep time: 10 minutes

½ cup of your favorite store-bought or homemade granola mix (any combination of oats, nuts, and dried fruit)

½ cup raspberries

½ cup blueberries, gently smashed with the back of a spoon

1 cup low-fat plain Greek-style yogurt

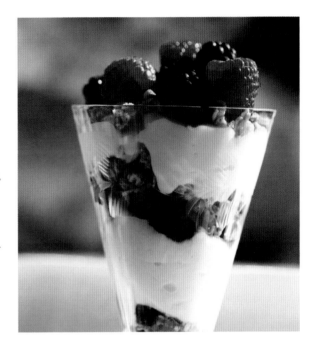

1 In a tall glass, layer about ⅓ granola, ⅓ banana, ⅓ blueberries, and ½ the yogurt.

2 Repeat layers, then top yogurt with remaining granola, banana, and blueberries.

Per serving: 468 calories, 13 g fat (5 g saturated), 71 g carbohydrates, 23 g protein, 7 g fiber, 10 mg cholesterol, 125 mg sodium

Spicy Egg-and-Cheese Scramble

The spicy seasoning in these waker-upper eggs will surely get you moving in no time. Serve with a slice of whole wheat toast to add a dose of high fiber.

Serves 1 ● PREP TIME: 15 minutes

2 eggs

1 teaspoon butter or olive oil (or cooking spray, if preferred)

1 tablespoon diced onion

1 tablespoon each diced green and red bell pepper

1 teaspoon garam masala, spicy steak seasoning, or combination of garlic pepper and red pepper flakes, to taste

¼ cup shredded sharp white cheddar cheese

1 In a small bowl, whisk eggs. Set aside.

2 Heat butter or olive oil in a heavy nonstick pan over medium heat. Add onions and peppers and sauté until tender. Add spicy seasoning to onion and pepper mix, then pour eggs into pan.

3 Stir eggs gently until just set. Sprinkle cheese over eggs; then, with a large spatula, transfer to a dish. Serve immediately.

Per serving: 284 calories, 22 g fat (12 g saturated), 4 g carbohydrates, 19 g protein, 1 g fiber, 463 mg cholesterol, 338 mg sodium

Curried Chicken Salad Sandwiches

This recipe is savory and sweet, high protein and low fat, and it's got that snappy apple and celery crunch. In other words, it's got it all!

MAKES 4 • PREP TIME: 10 minutes

¼ cup low-fat plain yogurt

2 tablespoons low-fat canola mayonnaise

1½ teaspoons curry powder

1 teaspoon honey

¼ teaspoon salt

2 cups chopped cooked chicken (8 ounces)

1 apple, cored and chopped

2 celery stalks, chopped

4 lettuce leaves

2 whole-grain pita breads
(8 inch/20 cm), halved

1 In a large bowl, whisk together yogurt, mayonnaise, curry powder, honey, and salt. Add chicken, apple, and celery.

2 Place a lettuce leaf in each pita half and fill with ¼ of the chicken salad.

Per serving (*1 filled half pocket*): 253 calories, 6 g total fat (1.6 g saturated), 27 g carbohydrates, 23 g protein, 4 g fiber, 53 mg cholesterol, 440 mg sodium

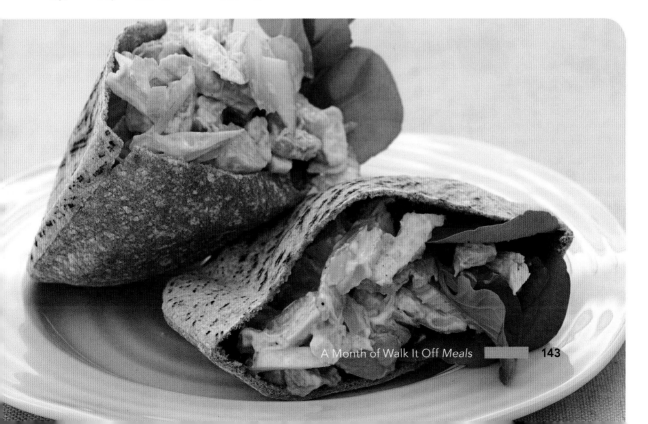

Cuban Bean Burritos

These quick-and-easy flavorful bundles are perfect to make the night before. Have one for lunch and freeze the rest for another day. Accompany them with some fresh pineapple for a refreshing citrus twist.

MAKES 4 ● PREP TIME: 30 minutes

½ cup long-grain white rice

2 tablespoons olive oil

1 cup chopped onion

4 garlic cloves, minced

1½ cups frozen mixed bell pepper strips

3 plum tomatoes, chopped

2 tablespoons red-wine vinegar

1 teaspoon dried oregano

1 can (15 ounces) black beans, drained but not rinsed

1 tablespoon grated fresh orange zest

4 burrito-size flour tortillas (8-inch/20-cm)

½ cup shredded sharp cheddar cheese (about 2 ounces)

1. Prepare rice according to package directions, omitting any fat.

2. Meanwhile, in a large pot, heat oil over medium-high heat. Add onion, garlic, and pepper strips. Cook, stirring occasionally, until vegetables begin to soften, about 5 minutes. Stir in tomatoes, vinegar, and oregano; cook for 2 minutes.

3. Add beans and reduce heat to medium. Cover and simmer until heated through and bubbly, about 10 minutes, stirring occasionally and lightly mashing some of the beans.

4. Remove pot from heat and stir in orange zest. Let stand for 3 minutes.

5. Heat flour tortillas according to package directions. Lay tortillas on a work surface. Spoon ½ cup rice onto each tortilla. Spoon ¾ cup bean mixture onto the rice. Sprinkle each with 2 tablespoons cheese.

6. Fold up the bottom quarter of each tortilla and roll away from you, tucking in the sides as you go. Set on serving plates, seam side down.

Per serving *(1 burrito):* 455 calories, 16 g total fat (4 g saturated), 64 g carbohydrates, 15 g protein, 7 g fiber, 15 mg cholesterol, 672 mg sodium, 228 mg calcium

Cold Sesame Noodles and Vegetables

The rainbow of crunchy veggies and hearty whole wheat pasta make this an especially satisfying meat-free meal.

SERVES 6 • PREP TIME: 20 minutes (plus 1 hour to chill)

8 ounces whole wheat linguine

⅓ cup cilantro leaves

2 tablespoons peanut butter

2 tablespoons reduced-sodium soy sauce

2½ teaspoons honey

1 tablespoon rice vinegar or cider vinegar

1 tablespoon dark sesame oil

2 cloves garlic, peeled

½ teaspoon salt

¼ teaspoon cayenne

2 carrots, slivered

1 red bell pepper, slivered

1 large stalk celery, slivered

2 scallions, slivered

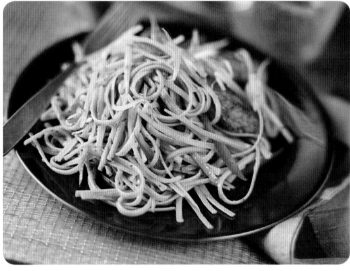

1 In a large pot of boiling water, cook linguine according to package directions. Drain, reserving ½ cup cooking water.

2 Meanwhile, in a food processor, combine cilantro, peanut butter, soy sauce, honey, vinegar, sesame oil, garlic, salt, and cayenne. Puree. Transfer to a large bowl.

3 Whisk in reserved pasta cooking water. Add linguine, carrots, bell pepper, celery, and scallions. Toss. Chill at least 1 hour before serving.

Per serving: 200 calories, 5.5 g total fat (1 g saturated), 33 g carbohydrates, 7 g protein, 6 g fiber, 0 mg cholesterol, 422 mg sodium

TIP For a hearty dinner, serve with grilled turkey burgers and garnish with chilled orange slices sprinkled with slivered almonds.

Pesto Tuna Wraps

The problem with most tuna wraps is that they're soggier than Seattle. This recipe offers two levels of protection: a pesto-flavored tuna salad without gloppy mayonnaise, and a shield of Romaine lettuce leaves between the salad and tortilla.

MAKES 4 ● PREP TIME: 10 MINUTES

2 cans (6 ounces each) water-packed solid white tuna, drained

½ cup prepared pesto

Juice of ½ lemon

¾ cup celery, finely chopped

¾ cup cucumber, seeded and finely chopped

1 cup grape tomatoes, halved

⅛ teaspoon salt

⅛ teaspoon black pepper

4 whole wheat tortillas (8-inch/20-cm)

3 cups torn romaine lettuce (small pieces)

1 In a medium bowl, combine tuna, pesto, oil, lemon juice, celery, cucumbers, tomatoes, salt, and black pepper.

2 For each wrap, start about 1 inch (2.5 cm) from bottom of tortilla and line the bottom third with ¾ cup lettuce. Top with tuna mixture.

3 Fold bottom of tortilla over filling, then fold each side in about 1 inch (2.5 cm). Roll firmly away from you. Cut each wrap in half on a diagonal.

Per serving: 366 calories, 15 g total fat (2 g saturated), 28 g protein, 4 g fiber, 40 mg cholesterol, 809 mg sodium, 125 mg calcium

Hummus and Pepper Jack Wraps

This wrap has become a standard vegetarian sandwich on menus everywhere. Creamy chickpea spread, spicy pepper Jack cheese, crunchy carrots, sweet bell peppers, juicy cucumbers.... What's not to love?

Makes 4 • PREP TIME: 15 MINUTES

1½ cups prepared hummus

4 whole wheat lavash (12-inch/30-cm)

½ cup shredded reduced-fat pepper Jack cheese

1 large red pepper, seeded and thinly sliced

1 cup shredded carrots

3 baby cucumbers, thinly sliced

2 scallions (white and green parts), chopped

2 tomatoes, thinly sliced

2 cups shredded romaine lettuce

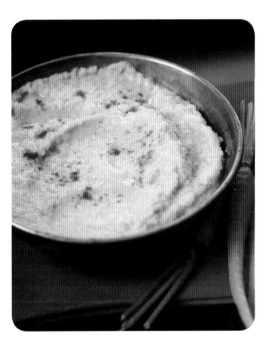

1 For each wrap, spread about ⅓ cup hummus over bottom half of lavash, stopping about 2 inches (5 cm) up from bottom. Layer with cheese, peppers, carrots, cucumbers, scallions, tomatoes, and lettuce.

2 Fold bottom of lavash over filling, then fold each side in about 1 inch (2.5 cm). Roll firmly away from you. Cut each wrap in half on a diagonal.

Per serving: 493 calories, 12 g total fat (3 g saturated), 18 g protein, 9 g fiber, 8 mg cholesterol, 724 mg sodium, 292 mg calcium

Lemony Lentil and Vegetable Salad

The lemon, goat cheese, and cilantro give this protein-rich salad a bright, tangy punch.

SERVES 4 • PREP TIME: 40 MINUTES

For the salad:

1 cup lentils, rinsed

1 garlic clove, peeled

Pinch ground cumin

1 slice lemon

1 small red onion, finely chopped

½ cup dried apricots, roughly chopped

3 small bell peppers (1 red, 1 yellow, and 1 green), seeded and cut into ¾-inch (2-cm) squares

¼ pound broccoli, broken into small florets

1 ounce reduced-fat goat cheese

2 tablespoons toasted sunflower seeds

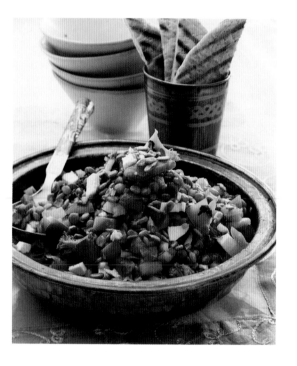

For the dressing:

Juice of 1 lemon

3 tablespoons olive oil

2 tablespoons finely chopped fresh cilantro

Salt and pepper, to taste

1 In a large saucepan, add lentils and cover with water. Bring to a boil, skimming off any scum. Add the garlic, cumin, and lemon slice, then reduce heat and simmer until lentils are tender, about 30 minutes.

2 Meanwhile, make the dressing: In a large salad bowl, whisk together the lemon juice, oil, cilantro, and salt and pepper to taste.

3 Drain lentils, discarding the lemon and garlic, and add to salad bowl. Toss gently to mix.

4 Add onion, apricots, peppers, and broccoli florets, and mix gently. Crumble goat cheese over top and scatter on sunflower seeds. Serve immediately.

Per serving: 361 calories, 15 g total fat (2 g saturated), 47 g carbohydrates, 15 g protein, 11 g fiber, 2 mg cholesterol, 116 mg sodium, 82 mg calcium

Quinoa and Chickpea Salad with Honey Lime Dressing

The high-fiber chickpeas in this recipe taste delicious combined with quinoa, a delicious gluten-free grain that's high in protein. For the best flavor, dress this salad and let it sit for 30 minutes before serving.

SERVES 4 ● PREP TIME: 25 MINUTES

For the salad:
2 cups low-sodium chicken stock

1⅓ cups quinoa, rinsed until water runs clear

1 can (8 ounces) chickpeas, rinsed and drained

1 cup chopped celery

1 cup roasted red peppers, chopped

⅓ cup finely chopped red onion

For the dressing:
Juice of 1 large lime

3 tablespoons extra-virgin olive oil

2 teaspoons honey

½ teaspoon salt

⅛ teaspoon ancho chile powder

1 tablespoon fresh cilantro, finely chopped

TIP Before using quinoa, it's critical to rinse it in a colander under cool water until the water runs clear. Rinsing removes the bitter-tasting saponins from the surface of the grains.

1 To make the salad, in a medium saucepan over high heat, bring chicken stock to a boil. Stir in quinoa and reduce heat to medium-low. Cover and simmer until most of the liquid has been absorbed (10–12 minutes). Turn off heat and let stand, covered, for 5 minutes. Fluff with a fork and set aside to cool.

2 Meanwhile, in a medium bowl, combine chickpeas, celery, roasted peppers, and onion. Add cooled quinoa and toss.

3 To make the dressing, in a small bowl, add lime juice and gradually whisk in oil in a steady stream. Whisk in honey, salt, and chile powder.

4 Pour dressing over salad and toss to coat. Divide among salad plates and scatter cilantro on top.

Per serving: 449 calories, 115 g total fat (2 g saturated), 4 g protein, 6 g fiber, 0 mg cholesterol, 794 mg sodium, 90 mg calcium

Black Bean Grapefruit Salad

The grapefruit in this hearty, fiber-rich bean salad adds an abundance of flavor and vitamin C.

SERVES 4 • PREP TIME: 15 MINUTES

TIP To keep grapefruit from tasting too bitter, cut off the rind and white pith just down to the flesh. To remove the segments, cut between the membranes in a V-shape. As you work around the grapefruit, scrape the juice from your cutting board into a cup and you'll end up with the 2 tablespoons required for the dressing.

For the dressing:

2 tablespoons fresh grapefruit juice

1 tablespoon fresh lime juice

3 tablespoons extra-virgin olive oil

1 teaspoon honey

¼ teaspoon salt

⅛ teaspoon black pepper

For the salad:

1 can (15 ounces) black beans, rinsed and drained

1 ruby red grapefruit, peeled, sectioned, and chopped

1 scallion (white and green parts), chopped

1 avocado, peeled, pitted, and chopped

4 large leaves romaine lettuce, torn

1 tablespoon cilantro, chopped

1 To make the dressing, in a medium bowl, combine grapefruit and lime juice. Slowly whisk in olive oil in a steady stream. Whisk in honey, salt, and pepper.

2 To make the salad, in the same bowl, add beans, grapefruit, and scallion; stir to combine. Gently fold in avocado.

3 Line four salad plates with lettuce. Top with salad mixture and scatter cilantro on top.

Per serving: 265 calories, 18 g total fat (3 g saturated), 5 g protein, 9 g fiber, o mg cholesterol, 335 mg sodium, 56 mg calcium

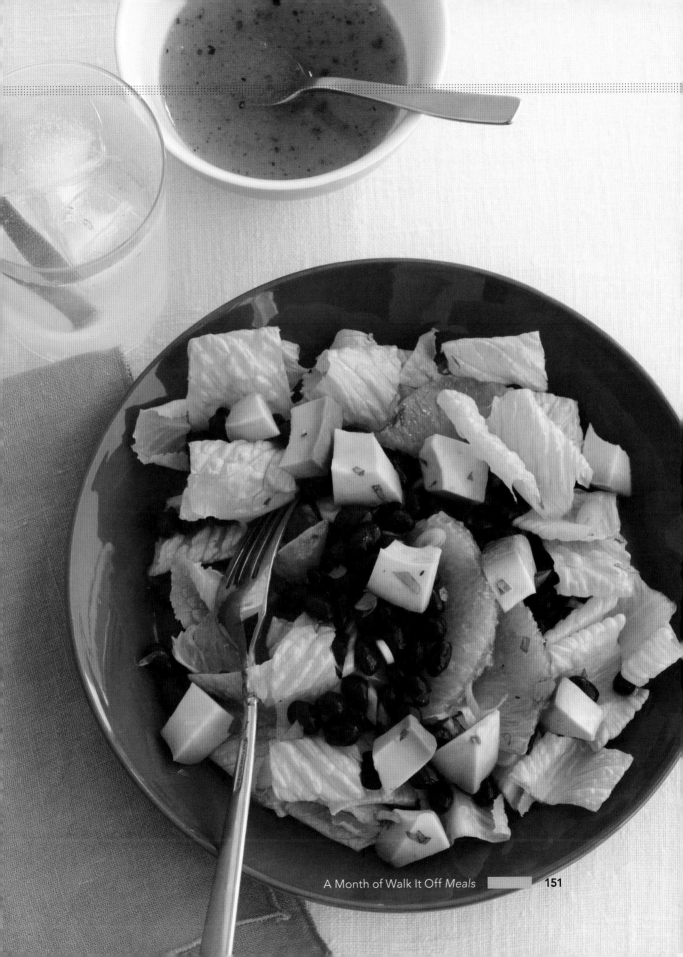

Feta Barley Salad with Citrus Dressing

Barley is one of the unsung heroes of the grain world. You can prepare it like risotto, simmer it as a hot breakfast cereal, or make it into a satisfying grain salad, as we've done here. Cranberries and orange complement this simple lunch salad.

SERVES 6 • PREP TIME: 25 MINUTES

> **TIP** Use sherry vinegar to add extra zip to any dressing. You can also sprinkle it on asparagus or add to stews for a touch of tangy sweetness.

For the salad:

1 cup quick-cooking barley

1 cup crumbled feta cheese

1 cup cucumber, seeded and chopped

1 cup green bell pepper, seeded and chopped

½ cup dried cranberries

⅓ cup red onion, finely chopped

For the dressing:

3 tablespoons fresh orange juice

1 tablespoon fresh lemon juice

¼ cup extra-virgin olive oil

Grated zest of 1 orange

¼ teaspoon salt

⅛ teaspoon freshly ground black pepper

2 tablespoons fresh mint, chopped

1 tablespoon fresh basil, chopped

1 To make the salad, cook barley according to package directions. Transfer to a medium bowl and let cool for 5 minutes.

2 Stir in cheese, cucumber, bell pepper, cranberries, and onion.

3 To make the dressing, in a small bowl, combine orange and lemon juice. Slowly whisk in oil in a steady stream; then whisk in orange zest, salt, and pepper.

4 Pour dressing over salad and toss to coat. Stir in mint and basil, reserving a few pinches for garnish.

Per serving: 313 calories, 15 g total fat (5 g saturated), 8 g protein, 7 g fiber, 22 mg cholesterol, 381 mg sodium, 151 mg calcium

Turkey Swiss Wraps

Watercress and English cucumbers give these quick-and-easy wraps a British flair.

Makes 4 • PREP TIME: 15 MINUTES

½ cup reduced-fat cream cheese

¼ cup fat-free Greek yogurt

2 tablespoons fresh basil, chopped

1 scallion (white and green parts), chopped

4 whole wheat tortillas (10-inch/25-cm)

12 ounces no-salt-added turkey breast, thinly sliced

6 ounces reduced-fat Swiss cheese, thinly sliced

1 cup shredded carrots

⅓ English cucumber or 2 small pickling cucumbers, thinly sliced

2 tomatoes, thinly sliced

1 bunch watercress, stem ends trimmed

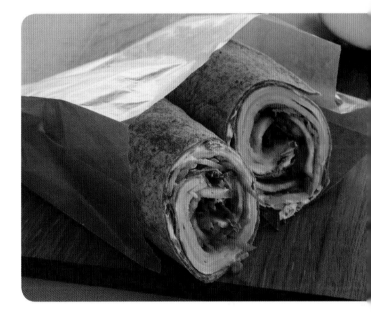

1 In a small bowl, mix cream cheese, yogurt, basil, and scallions.

2 For each wrap, spread about 3 tablespoons cream cheese mixture evenly over a tortilla. Starting about 1 inch (2.5 cm) up from bottom, line the bottom third of a tortilla with turkey, cheese, carrots, cucumber, tomatoes, and watercress.

3 Fold the bottom of the tortilla over the filling, then fold in each side about 1 inch (2.5 cm). Roll firmly away from you. Cut each wrap in half on a diagonal.

Per serving: 385 calories, 9 g total fat (5 g saturated), 45 g protein, 3 g fiber, 102 mg cholesterol, 460 mg sodium, 555 mg calcium

TIP Look for long, skinny English cucumbers wrapped in plastic in the produce aisle. They have a thinner skin plus fewer and less-bitter seeds than hothouse cukes. You can also use small thin-skinned pickling cucumbers or Persian cukes.

Barley, Black Bean, and Avocado Salad

Every ingredient in this salad packs a seriously-good-for-you punch. The beans and barley alone give you half your daily requirement of cholesterol-lowering, belly-filling fiber.

SERVES 4 • PREP TIME: 25 minutes

1 cup carrot juice

½ teaspoon thyme

½ teaspoon salt

⅛ teaspoon cayenne

½ cup quick-cooking barley

3 tablespoons fresh lemon juice

1 tablespoon olive oil

1 can (19 ounces) black beans, rinsed and drained

1 cup diced tomatoes

½ cup diced avocado

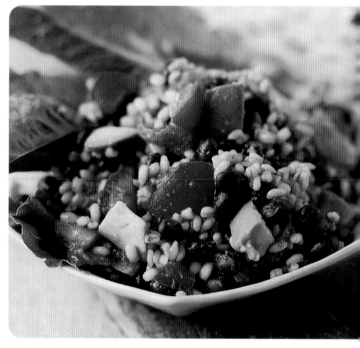

1 In medium saucepan, combine carrot juice, thyme, salt, and cayenne. Bring to a boil over medium heat; add barley and reduce to a simmer. Cover and cook until barley is tender, about 15 minutes.

2 Meanwhile, in a large bowl, whisk together lemon juice and oil. Transfer barley and any liquid remaining in pan to bowl with lemon-juice mixture. Toss to coat.

3 Add beans and tomatoes and toss to combine. Add avocado and gently toss once more. Serve at room temperature or chilled. For best flavor, remove from refrigerator 20 minutes before serving.

Per serving: 259 calories, 7 g total fat (1.4 g saturated), 42 g carbohydrates, 10 g protein, 11 g fiber, 0 mg cholesterol, 461 mg sodium

Sesame Chicken Wraps

Light sesame-ginger dressing supplies the flavor here. Look for it among the bottled salad dressings in your grocery store.

MAKES 4 • PREP TIME: 30 MINUTES (PLUS 2–3 HOURS FOR MARINATING)

2 to 3 boneless skinless chicken breasts (about a pound),
pounded to an even ½-inch (1.5-cm) thickness

⅔ cup light sesame-ginger dressing

4 whole wheat lavash (12-inch/30-cm)

2 cups shredded iceberg lettuce

1 cup shredded carrots

1 cup snow peas, cut lengthwise into thin strips

1 can (8 ounces) sliced water chestnuts, drained and cut into slivers

2 scallions (white and green parts), chopped

1 teaspoon toasted sesame seeds

1 teaspoon toasted sesame oil

1 Combine chicken and dressing in a 1-gallon zipper-seal bag. Press out the air, seal, and refrigerate for 2 to 3 hours.

2 Transfer chicken to a plate and pour marinade into small saucepan. Boil marinade over medium heat for 5 minutes. Set aside to cool.

3 Bring a grill or large grill pan to medium-high heat. Add chicken and cook until juices run clear, about 3 to 4 minutes per side. Set aside to cool.

4 To make each wrap, start about 1 inch (2.5 cm) up from bottom and line bottom third of lavash with about ½ cup lettuce. Top with the carrots, snow peas, water chestnuts, scallions, and sesame seeds.

5 Slice chicken into thin strips and arrange over filling. Stir sesame oil into boiled and cooled marinade. Drizzle about 2 tablespoons of the mixture over chicken.

6 Fold bottom of lavash over filling, then fold in each side about 1 inch (2.5 cm). Roll firmly away from you. Cut each wrap in half on a diagonal.

Per serving: 478 calories, 6 g total fat (1 g saturated), 36 g protein, 6 g fiber, 66 mg cholesterol, 790 mg sodium, 40 mg calcium

TIP To easily cut the water chestnuts into slivers, line them up in a vertical column on your cutting board, then slice down the column every ¼ inch (1 cm) or so.

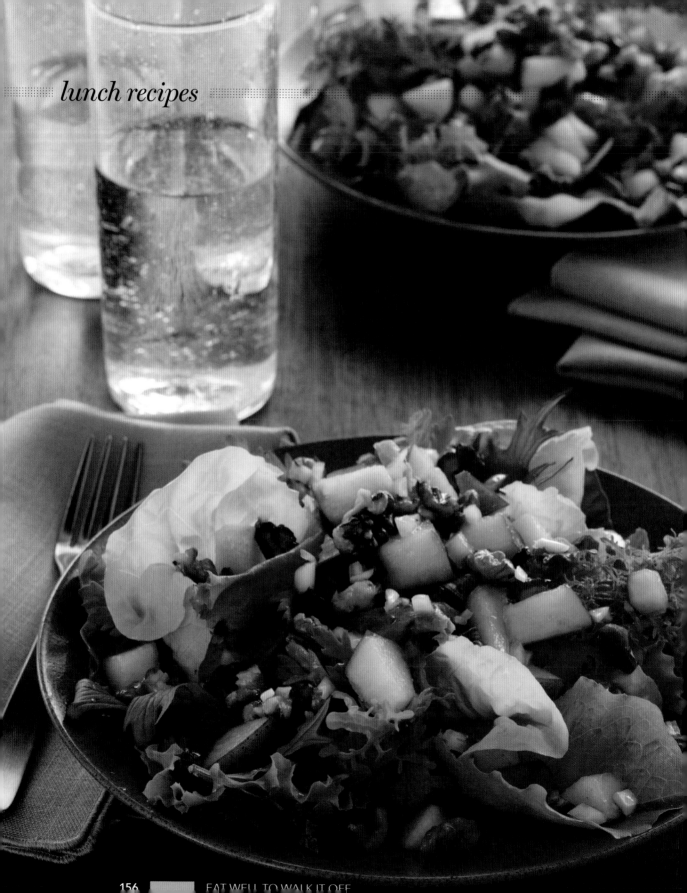

Lettuces with Pears, Dates, and Manchego Cheese

Utterly simple yet supremely satisfying, this salad also makes a fabulous presentation. And it's quick, too.

MAKES 4 ● PREP TIME: 10 MINUTES

4 ounces baby leaf lettuces, such as oak leaf, lollo rosso, and frisée

3 ripe Bosc pears, cored and finely chopped

2 teaspoons lemon juice

6 pitted dates, finely chopped

2 tablespoons walnuts, chopped

1 small shallot, minced

2 teaspoons sherry vinegar

5 teaspoons extra-virgin olive oil

½ teaspoon coarse salt

⅛ teaspoon ground black pepper

8 to 10 thin shavings Manchego cheese (about 2 ounces total)

1 Divide lettuces among four salad plates.

2 Toss the pears with the lemon juice and divide among the plates along with the dates, walnuts, and shallots.

3 Sprinkle evenly with the vinegar, oil, salt, and black pepper.

4 Top with Manchego cheese.

Per serving: 256 calories, 12 g total fat (3 g saturated), 10 mg cholesterol, 5 g protein, 6 g fiber, 488 mg sodium, 97 mg calcium

TIP To help keep sticky dates from adhering to your knife blade while chopping, lightly coat the blade with cooking spray first.

Broccoli and Cheese Calzones

The raisins, curry powder, and Dijon mustard give these tasty bundles a savory kick. And the reduced-fat cheeses provide just as much protein, vitamins, and minerals as their full-fat counterparts.

MAKES 6 ● PREP TIME: 40 minutes

1 cup shredded reduced-fat cheddar cheese

½ cup shredded fat-free mozzarella

½ cup raisins

2 tablespoons Dijon mustard

1 tablespoon curry powder

¾ teaspoon pepper

¼ teaspoon salt

1 package (10 ounces) frozen chopped broccoli, thawed and drained

1 pound frozen pizza dough, thawed

1 Preheat oven to 450°F (232°C). Line large baking sheet with parchment paper.

2 In a medium bowl, combine cheddar, mozzarella, raisins, mustard, curry powder, pepper, and salt. Add drained broccoli and stir to combine.

3 Divide pizza dough into 6 portions. Roll each portion out to a 7-inch (18-cm) round. Spoon ½ cup cheese mixture onto half of round, leaving ½-inch (1.5-cm) border. Fold top over and press edges together to seal. Repeat with remaining dough and filling. Place on baking sheet.

4 Bake 22 to 25 minutes or until crust is golden brown and crisp. Let stand 10 minutes before serving.

Per serving: 325 calories, 6.5 g total fat (1 g saturated), 50 g carbohydrates, 18 g protein, 4 g fiber, 11 mg cholesterol, 881 mg sodium

Grilled Jamaican Jerk Chicken

The saucy seasoning mixture is a uniquely Caribbean blend of spicy, sweet, and hot and adds spark to Jamaican-style "jerk" meats and poultry. We've added bell pepper, pineapple, and scallions and, to spare tender palates, substituted a pickled jalapeño for the more traditional and extremely hot Scotch Bonnet chilies. Serve with brown rice pilaf, and slice a mango for dessert.

SERVES 4 • PREP TIME: 45 MINUTES (PLUS 1 HOUR FOR MARINATING)

1 tablespoon ground allspice

4 cloves garlic, minced

1 tablespoon minced fresh ginger

1 large pickled jalapeño pepper, minced

¼ cup white wine vinegar

1½ tablespoons light brown sugar

1½ tablespoons olive oil

1¼ teaspoons black pepper

¾ teaspoon salt

4 boneless, skinless chicken breast halves (5 ounces each)

8 scallions

2 large red bell peppers, cut into 32 chunks

Canned pineapple chunks (about 1½ cups)

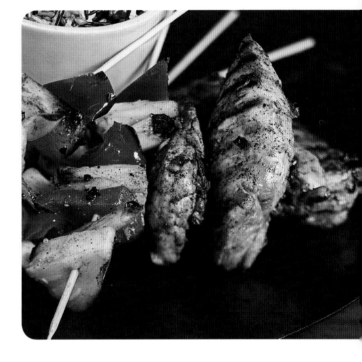

1 In a large bowl, combine allspice, garlic, ginger, jalapeño, vinegar, brown sugar, oil, black pepper, and salt. Measure out 2 tablespoons of mixture and set aside.

2 In same bowl, add chicken and turn to coat on all sides. Refrigerate for 1 hour. (Don't marinate longer than 1 hour or ginger and vinegar will start to break down the fiber of the chicken.)

3 Trim scallions, leaving off just a small portion of tender green. Cut each scallion into 3 pieces.

4 Preheat grill to medium. On each of 8 long skewers, alternately thread 3 pieces scallion, 4 pieces bell pepper, and 3 pieces pineapple.

5 Lift chicken from marinade and place on grill. Brush reserved 2 tablespoons spice mixture over skewers and place on grill. Grill, turning chicken and skewers once, until chicken is cooked through and vegetables are crisp tender, 5 to 10 minutes for skewers, 10 to 15 minutes for chicken.

Per serving: 302 calories, 7.5 g total fat (1.5 g saturated), 25 g carbohydrates, 35 g protein, 4 g fiber, 82 mg cholesterol, 558 mg sodium

BLT Pasta Salad

Switching it up with colorful pasta gives a whole new appreciation for the ingredients of this all-time favorite sandwich. Using turkey bacon leans it down, while the watercress adds a peppery bite.

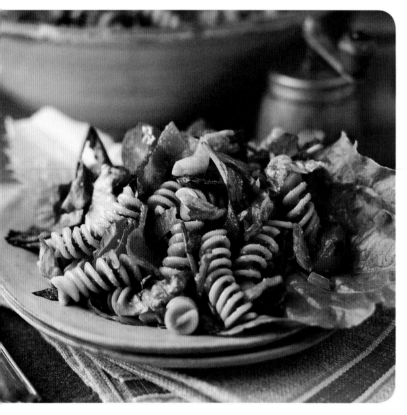

SERVES 4 ● PREP TIME: 30 MINUTES

12 ounces tricolor fusilli

2 teaspoons olive oil

5 slices turkey bacon, cut crosswise into ½-inch (1.5-cm) strips

1 large onion, cut into ½-inch (1.5-cm) chunks

3 cloves garlic, minced

1 pint red and/or yellow cherry tomatoes, halved

¾ teaspoon salt

8 cups coarsely chopped watercress or shredded romaine lettuce, or a combination

⅓ cup grated Parmesan cheese

1 In large pot of boiling water, cook fusilli according to package directions. Drain, reserving ½ cup cooking water.

2 Meanwhile, in a large nonstick skillet over medium heat, heat oil. Add bacon, onion, and garlic. Cook, stirring frequently, until onion is golden, about 7 minutes.

3 Add tomatoes and salt to skillet and cook until tomatoes begin to soften but still hold their shape, about 5 minutes.

4 Place greens in large bowl. In skillet, add reserved cooking water to tomatoes and bring to a boil. Pour hot tomato mixture over greens. Add pasta and Parmesan and toss to combine.

Per serving: 410 calories, 10 g total fat (2.5 g saturated), 65 g carbohydrates, 20 g protein, 7 g fiber, 22 mg cholesterol, 876 mg sodium

Chicken with Apples and Calvados

The tart apples, apple juice, Calvados, and bit of cream give this high-protein dish a rich flair.

SERVES 6 • PREP TIME: 30 MINUTES

2 medium shallots, finely chopped

2 tart apples, peeled and cut into ¼-inch (1-cm) slices

1 cup apple juice

¾ cup reduced-sodium chicken broth

1 tablespoon Calvados, applejack, or apple juice

¼ cup all-purpose flour

½ teaspoon salt

½ teaspoon freshly ground black pepper

4 boneless, skinless chicken breast halves (5 ounces each)

2 tablespoons heavy cream

1 Lightly coat a large, heavy nonstick skillet with cooking spray and set over medium-high heat. Sauté shallots until soft, about 2 minutes. Add apples and sauté until lightly browned, about 3 minutes. Add apple juice, broth, and Calvados. Cook, stirring, until apples are tender, about 5 minutes. Transfer to medium bowl. Wipe skillet clean.

2 Meanwhile, on a sheet of waxed paper, combine flour, salt, and pepper. Coat chicken breasts with seasoned flour, pressing with your hands so flour adheres and chicken is flattened evenly.

3 Lightly coat skillet again with cooking spray and set over medium-high heat. Cook chicken until browned and almost cooked through, about 3 minutes on each side. Add apple mixture and any juices and bring to a boil. Reduce heat and simmer 2 minutes. Stir in cream and remove from heat.

Per serving: 300 calories, 5 g total fat (2 g saturated), 26 g carbohydrates, 35 g protein, 2 g fiber, 93 mg cholesterol, 402 mg sodium

MAKE-IT-SNAPPY DESSERTS

No need to make a big old Lady Baltimore cake to satisfy your dessert cravings. Instead, keep it natural and simple. Here are five quick-and-easy dessert ideas you can adapt to your personal fruit preferences that will help keep your sweet tooth under control:

• Frozen banana on a Popsicle stick

• Cup of frozen watermelon balls, grapes, or pineapple chunks drizzled with yogurt

• Homemade fruit smoothie ice pop

• Roasted pear drizzled with honey

• Grilled peach with a spoonful of raspberry jam

Chicken Kabobs with Cherry Tomatoes

Chicken breast is very low in calories. To give it more flavor, we marinate it in a lemony vinaigrette for two days. What a revelation! The chicken appears white from the acidity of the marinade and develops a delicious taste and texture.

MAKES 8 • PREP TIME: 20 MINUTES (PLUS 2 DAYS FOR MARINATING)

½ cup olive oil

Juice of 2 lemons

3 tablespoons white wine vinegar

6 bay leaves, finely crumbled or chopped

6 large garlic cloves, minced

2 teaspoons salt

1 tablespoon dried oregano

2 teaspoons dried basil

2 teaspoons dried thyme

1 teaspoon ground black pepper

2½ pounds boneless skinless chicken breast, cut into 1½-inch (4-cm) cubes

1 pint cherry tomatoes

1 In a large zipper-seal bag, whisk together oil, lemon juice, vinegar, bay leaves, garlic, salt, oregano, basil, thyme, and pepper. Into a small bowl, pour ¼ cup marinade, cover, and refrigerate.

2 Drop the chicken into the zipper-seal bag, press out air, seal, and refrigerate for 2 days. If necessary to "melt" the olive oil (which can solidify in the fridge), remove bag from refrigerator a couple times a day, shaking bag to redistribute the marinade, then return to refrigerator.

3 About 20 minutes before grilling, remove chicken and bowl of reserved marinade from refrigerator. Heat grill to medium-high.

4 Meanwhile, remove chicken from marinade, reserving the marinade in the bag. Thread chicken and tomatoes alternately on 8 large skewers or 16 small ones.

5 Grill skewers until chicken is nicely browned and no longer pink in the center, 8 to 10 minutes, turning often and drizzling with bagged marinade during first 5 to 7 minutes. Avoid overcooking; chicken should be very moist and register about 165°F (74°C) on an instant-read thermometer.

6 Transfer to plates and drizzle on reserved marinade.

Per serving: 300 calories, 15 g total fat (2 g saturated), 6 g carbohydrates, 34 g protein, 1 g fiber, 82 mg cholesterol, 679 mg sodium

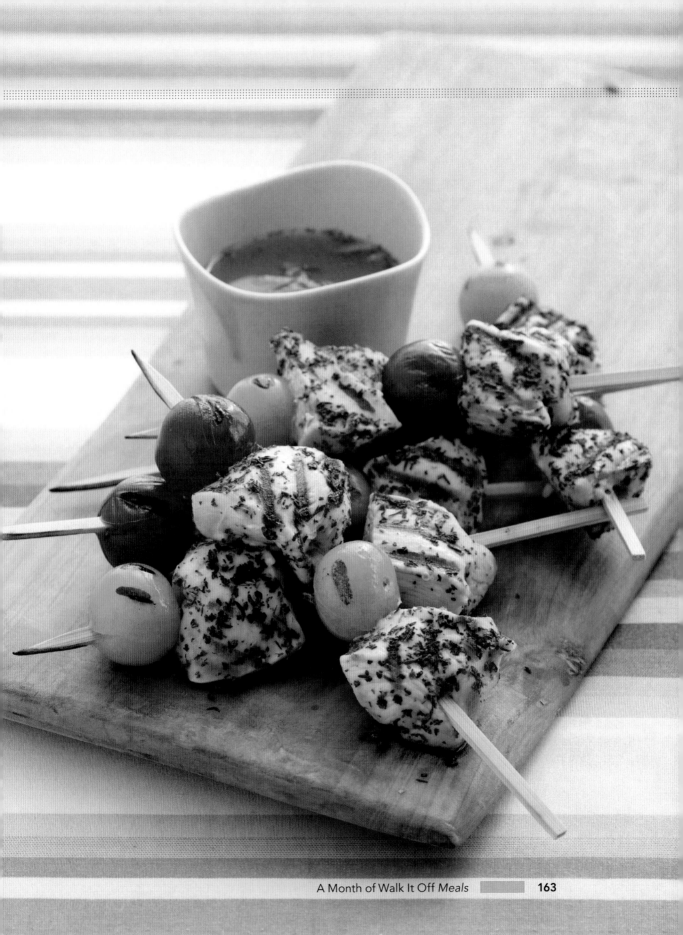

Asian Chicken Salad

It's hard to believe this salad's creamy, garlicky peanut dressing is loaded with goodness. The protein and "good fat" in the peanut butter help boost energy and stabilize blood sugar.

SERVES 4 • PREP TIME: 20 MINUTES

1 pound romaine lettuce, finely shredded

4 ounces snow peas

1 can (20 ounces) lychees, drained and cut in half

1 large navel orange, peeled and cut into sections

1 red plum, pitted and sliced

4 scallions, thinly sliced

12 ounces boneless, skinless chicken breast halves

$\frac{1}{3}$ cup nonfat mayonnaise

3 tablespoons creamy peanut butter

1 garlic clove, minced

TIP For a heartier meal serve over room-temperature Asian noodles, which can be found at your local grocery store or Asian market.

1 In large salad bowl, add romaine. Trim snow peas and remove strings with fingers. Cut peas in half on the diagonal and add to salad bowl, along with lychees, orange, plum, and scallions. Toss to mix.

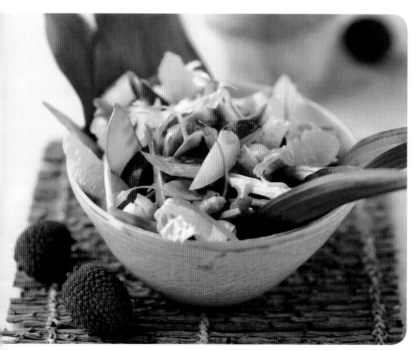

2 Coat nonstick ridged grill pan with cooking spray and set over medium-high heat until hot, about 2 minutes. Grill chicken breasts until cooked through, about 4 minutes on each side.

3 Meanwhile, in a small measuring cup, whisk mayonnaise, peanut butter, and garlic until dressing is blended. Cut chicken into thin slices diagonally and add to salad bowl. Right before serving, drizzle salad with dressing and toss to coat.

Per serving: 378 calories, 9 g total fat (2.5 g saturated), 53 g carbohydrates, 27 g protein, 7 g fiber, 49 mg cholesterol, 378 mg sodium

Santa Fe Stuffed Peppers

Here, roasted whole bell peppers are packed with a southwestern medley of rice, beef, beans, and salsa. They're spiced up, just like chiles rellenos—without the fuss or the fat.

MAKES 4 • PREP TIME: 40 MINUTES

4 large red, yellow, or green bell peppers

1 cup reduced-sodium chicken broth

1 cup instant brown rice

1 large onion, chopped

8 ounces lean (95%) ground beef

1 cup chunky salsa

½ cup drained, rinsed canned black beans

¼ teaspoon freshly ground black pepper

⅓ cup shredded nonfat cheddar cheese

1 Preheat broiler. Line broiler pan with foil, leaving 2-inch (5-cm) overhang. Fit with slotted rack. Arrange whole bell peppers on rack and place about 8 inches (20 cm) from heat. Broil, turning about every 4 minutes, until skin is charred and blistered on all sides, about 10 minutes. Slide peppers onto foil; crimp tightly to close. Let stand until tender, about 10 minutes.

2 Meanwhile, in a small saucepan over high heat, bring chicken broth to a boil. Stir in rice and simmer 5 minutes. Remove from heat, cover, and let stand 5 minutes. Drain any liquid that remains, then set aside, keeping rice warm.

3 Peel off dark skin from peppers with small paring knife, keeping stems intact. Make a slit along one side of peppers to create an opening and carefully remove seeds with small spoon.

4 Set large nonstick skillet over medium-high heat. Sauté onion and beef until onion is soft and beef is no longer pink, about 7 minutes. Stir in rice, salsa, beans, and black pepper. Spoon rice mixture into bell peppers. Return peppers to broiler pan. Sprinkle with cheddar and broil until cheese melts, about 1 minute.

Per serving: 284 calories, 5 g total fat (1.5 g saturated), 39 g carbohydrates, 23 g protein, 7 g fiber, 28 mg cholesterol, 804 mg sodium

Sizzling Beef Fajitas

This Mexican fiesta-on-a-plate stays within your calorie budget by using sirloin (a low-fat cut) and plenty of veggies. Serve smoking hot from the broiler. It's a treat for the family and also ideal party fare.

MAKES 4 • PREP TIME: 30 MINUTES

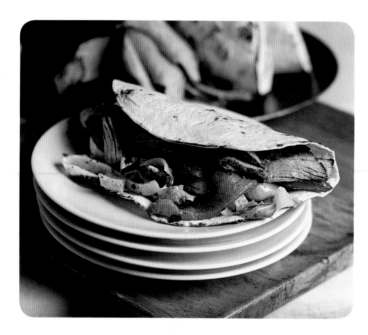

¼ cup fresh lime juice

1 teaspoon chili powder

¾ teaspoon oregano

¾ teaspoon ground coriander

¼ teaspoon black pepper

12 ounces well-trimmed beef sirloin

2 large onions, thickly sliced

2 large red bell peppers, cut lengthwise into flat panels

¼ cup minced cilantro

4 flour tortillas (8-inch/20-cm)

4 cups shredded romaine lettuce

¼ cup fat-free sour cream

1 In medium bowl, combine lime juice, chili powder, oregano, coriander, and black pepper and set aside.

2 In a shallow bowl, place beef and spoon 2 tablespoons of lime mixture on top; turn to coat. Let stand.

3 Meanwhile, preheat broiler. Spray broiler pan with nonstick cooking spray. Place onions and pepper pieces, skin-side up, on broiler pan. Broil 4 inches (10 cm) from heat until peppers are charred and onions are golden brown, about 10 minutes. Remove and, when cool enough to handle, peel peppers and thickly slice. Add peppers and onions to lime juice mixture. Add cilantro and toss.

4 Broil beef until done to medium, about 8 minutes, turning over midway. Let stand 5 minutes before thinly slicing. Broil tortillas until lightly browned, about 15 seconds per side.

5 Place beef, peppers and onions, lettuce, sour cream, and flour tortillas in serving containers for a self-serve buffet.

Per serving: 379 calories, 9 g total fat (3 g saturated), 45 g carbohydrates, 29 g protein, 6 g fiber, 63 mg cholesterol, 319 mg sodium

Southwestern Shepherd's Pie

Extra-lean ground beef combined with fiber-rich kidney beans creates an indulgent treat that won't break the calorie bank. Serve with a tossed salad.

SERVES 4 • PREP TIME: 1 HOUR

2 teaspoons olive oil

4 scallions, thinly sliced

6 cloves garlic, minced

1 large green bell pepper, chopped

6 ounces extra-lean ground sirloin

1 tablespoon chili powder

1½ teaspoons ground coriander

1½ teaspoons ground cumin

1½ cups canned tomatoes, chopped with their juice

1 can (15 ounces) red kidney beans, rinsed and drained

1½ pounds all-purpose potatoes, peeled and thinly sliced

¾ teaspoon salt

⅓ cup chopped cilantro

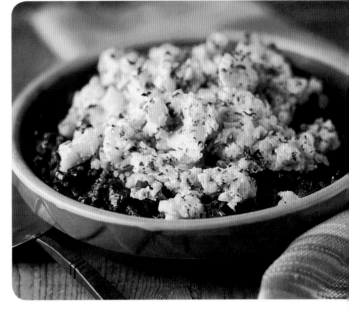

1 Heat oil in large nonstick skillet over low heat. Add scallions and half the garlic and cook, stirring frequently until tender, about 2 minutes. Add bell pepper, increase heat to medium, and cook, stirring until pepper is crisp tender, about 5 minutes.

2 Stir in beef, chili powder, coriander, and cumin. Cook, stirring occasionally to break up beef, until beef is no longer pink, about 2 minutes. Stir in tomatoes and beans and bring to a boil. Reduce to a simmer, cover, and cook until mixture is thick and flavorful, about 10 minutes.

3 Meanwhile, in medium saucepan, boil water and add potatoes and remaining garlic. Cook until tender, about 10 minutes.

4 Reserve ¼ cup of potato cooking liquid and set aside in a small bowl. Drain off remaining liquid and keep potatoes and garlic in pan. Return reserved cooking liquid to pan along with salt. With potato masher, mash potatoes and garlic until not quite smooth, leaving some texture. Stir in cilantro.

5 Preheat oven to 425°F (218°C). Spoon meat mixture into 9-inch (23-cm) deep-dish pie plate. Spoon mashed potatoes over top. (Recipe can be made ahead up to this point. Cover and refrigerate. Return to room temperature before baking.) Bake until filling is bubbling, about 15 minutes.

Per serving: 280 calories, 7.5 g total fat (2 g saturated), 42 g carbohydrates, 15 g protein, 6 g fiber, 15 mg cholesterol, 974 mg sodium

Asian BBQ Beef with Water Chestnut Salad

A light citrus-sesame-soy marinade flavors naturally low-fat flank steak in this dish inspired by Southeast Asian street food. The water chestnut salad and brown rice add waist-friendly fiber.

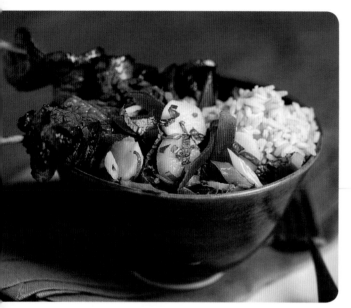

SERVES 4 • PREP TIME: 30 MINUTES (PLUS 1 HOUR FOR MARINATING)

10 ounces well-trimmed flank steak

½ cup orange juice

2 tablespoons reduced-sodium soy sauce

2 teaspoons dark sesame oil

1 tablespoon plus 1 teaspoon light brown sugar

1 teaspoon ground ginger

¼ teaspoon red pepper flakes

1 red bell pepper, slivered

2 scallions, thinly sliced

2 tablespoons chopped fresh mint

½ teaspoon salt

1 can (8 ounces) sliced water chestnuts, drained

1 cup brown rice

1 Thinly slice flank steak across the grain to make 8 thin slices.

2 Combine ¼ cup orange juice, soy sauce, sesame oil, 1 tablespoon brown sugar, ginger, and ⅛ teaspoon red pepper flakes in shallow bowl. Add beef slices, tossing to coat. Cover and refrigerate for 1 hour or up to overnight.

3 Meanwhile, to make the salad, combine bell pepper, scallions, mint, and salt with remaining ¼ cup orange juice, 1 teaspoon brown sugar, and ⅛ teaspoon red pepper flakes. Add water chestnuts, toss to combine, and refrigerate until serving time.

4 Cook brown rice according to package directions. Fluff with fork.

5 Preheat broiler. Lift meat from its marinade and thread onto eight 12-inch (30-cm) skewers. Place skewers on broiler pan and broil 4 inches (10 cm) from heat, brushing with marinade after 2 minutes. Turn skewers over and broil 2 minutes. Serve skewers on rice with water chestnut salad.

Per serving: 370 calories, 9.5 g total fat (3 g saturated), 51 g carbohydrates, 20 g protein, 4 g fiber, 37 mg cholesterol, 614 mg sodium

Soy-Marinated Pork Tenderloin

Pork tenderloin is one of the leanest meats of all, but this delicious marinade is so rich in flavor, you'll think you're breaking the calorie bank.

SERVES 6 ● PREP TIME: 30 MINUTES (PLUS 2 HOURS FOR MARINATING)

¾ cup reduced-sodium soy sauce

Grated zest and juice of 1½ lemons

1½ tablespoons honey

1 tablespoon canola oil

1 tablespoon toasted sesame oil

4 large garlic cloves, minced

1 tablespoon minced fresh ginger

4 scallions (green and white parts), trimmed and chopped

Pinch of cayenne pepper

2 pork tenderloins, 12 to 16 ounces each

> **TIP** Pork tenderloin is covered with a thin, shiny membrane called the silverskin. If left on, the silverskin can cause the tenderloin to curl up during cooking. Remove the silverskin by grabbing it at the thick end of the meat and separate it from the meat with a small knife.

1 Combine soy sauce, lemon zest, lemon juice, honey, canola oil, sesame oil, garlic, ginger, scallions, and ground red pepper in a large zipper-seal bag. Pour ¼ cup of the marinade into a bowl, cover, and refrigerate. Pour half of the remaining marinade into another large zipper-seal bag. Drop one tenderloin into each bag, press out the air, seal, and refrigerate for 2 to 3 hours.

2 Once tenderloins finish marinating, heat a grill to medium-high.

3 Remove tenderloins from marinade and pat dry with paper towels. Discard marinade. Let meat rest at room temperature as grill heats up. Remove bowl of reserved marinade from refrigerator.

4 Grill tenderloins until browned all over, 2 to 3 minutes on each of the four sides, brushing now and then with the reserved marinade. Reduce heat under tenderloins to medium-low (on a gas grill) or move tenderloins to a lower-heat area (on a charcoal grill). Cover and continue cooking over medium-low heat until meat is just firm when poked and an instant-read thermometer registers 145°F (63°C), about another 2 to 3 minutes on each of the four sides; brush with reserved marinade now and then.

5 Transfer to a platter, cover loosely with foil, and let rest for 5 minutes before slicing.

Per serving: 222 calories, 9 g total fat (2 g saturated), 7 g carbohydrates, 26 g protein, 1 g fiber, 74 mg cholesterol, 621 mg sodium

Green Pork Chili

People who love cilantro will love this dish, with its distinctive southwestern flavor.

SERVES 4 • PREP TIME: 30 MINUTES

2 tablespoons olive oil

1 pound pork tenderloin, cut into 1-inch (2.5-cm) chunks

2 tablespoons flour

6 scallions, thinly sliced

3 cloves garlic, minced

1 large green bell pepper, cut into ½-inch (1.5-cm) chunks

1 pickled jalapeño pepper, finely chopped

1 can (4½ ounces) chopped mild green chilies

1½ cups packed cilantro sprigs, chopped

¾ teaspoon salt

½ teaspoon ground coriander

1½ cups frozen peas, thawed

2 tablespoons fresh lime juice

1 red bell pepper, slivered

1 Preheat oven to 350°F (177°C). In a nonstick Dutch oven or flameproof casserole, heat oil over medium heat. Dredge pork in flour, shaking off excess. Add pork to oil and sauté for 4 minutes, or until golden brown. With a slotted spoon, transfer the pork to a plate.

2 Add scallions and garlic to pan and cook for 1 minute, or until scallions are tender. Add green bell pepper and jalapeño and cook for 4 minutes, or until bell pepper is crisp tender. Stir in mild green chilies, half the cilantro, salt, ground coriander, and 1¼ cups water; bring to a boil.

3 Return pork to pan. Cover, place in the oven, and bake for 25 minutes, or until pork is tender.

4 Stir in peas, lime juice, and remaining cilantro. Re-cover and let stand for 3 minutes. Serve topped with the red bell pepper.

Per serving: 306 calories, 13 g total fat (3 g saturated), 19 g carbohydrates, 28 g protein, 4.3 g fiber, 75 mg cholesterol, 810 mg sodium

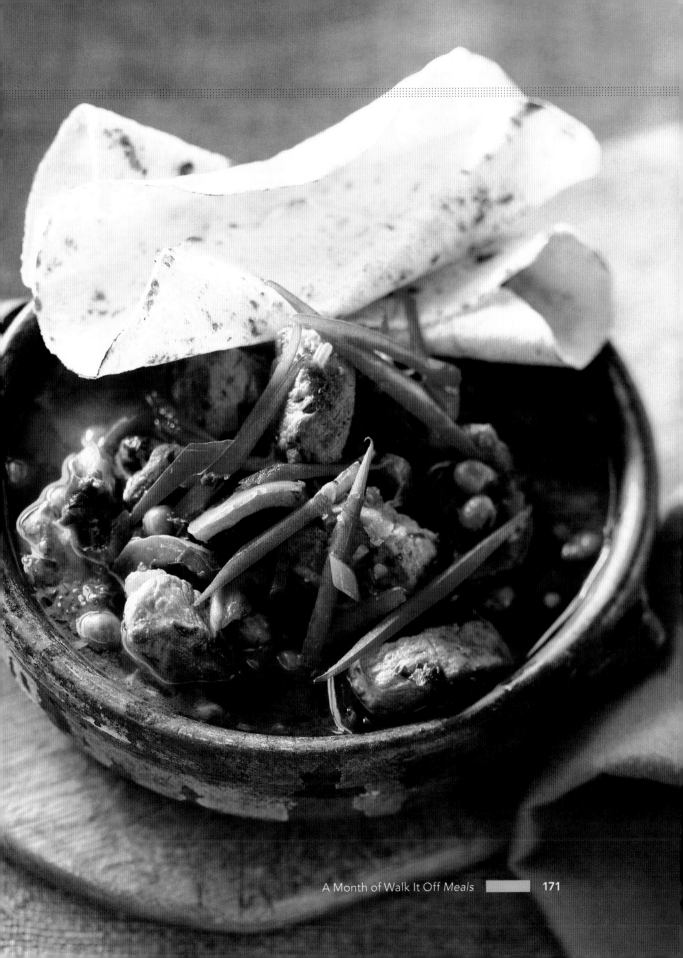

Caribbean Seafood Curry Stew

A riot of flavors, from ginger and curry to hot pepper and lime, make halibut and shrimp come alive as never before.

SERVES 4 • PREP TIME: 35 minutes

2 teaspoons olive oil

6 thin scallions, finely chopped

1 yellow bell pepper, coarsely chopped

1 tablespoon minced fresh ginger

1½ teaspoons curry powder

¼ to ½ teaspoon hot red pepper flakes

¼ teaspoon ground allspice

2 tablespoons reduced-sodium soy sauce

1½ tablespoons brown sugar

¼ teaspoon salt

1 can (14 ounces) reduced-fat coconut milk

3 plum tomatoes, quartered lengthwise and seeded

½ pound halibut steaks, skin removed and cut into 2-inch (5-cm) chunks

½ pound medium shrimp, peeled and deveined

2 tablespoons chopped cilantro

1 tablespoon lime juice

> **TIP** To make this dish ahead of time, follow the directions through cooking the seafood in step 2. Cool to room temperature, then refrigerate for up to one day. Reheat, then stir in cilantro and lime juice.

1 In large saucepan over medium heat, heat oil. Add scallions, bell pepper, and ginger. Sauté until softened, 5 minutes. Add curry powder, pepper flakes to taste, and allspice. Sauté 2 minutes. Stir in soy sauce, brown sugar, and salt. Stir in coconut milk and tomatoes. Gently simmer, uncovered, 15 minutes.

2 Add halibut and shrimp to stew mixture. Gently simmer, uncovered, just until fish is cooked through, 5 to 8 minutes. Stir in cilantro and lime juice and serve.

Per serving: 223 calories, 9 g total fat (4 g saturated), 17 g carbohydrates, 22 g protein, 2 g fiber, 99 mg cholesterol, 605 mg sodium

Baltimore Seafood Cakes

These crab-and-shrimp cakes are spiced with mustard, Worcestershire sauce, and a little cayenne pepper. But the secret ingredient is ground almonds mixed right into the cakes before being coated in breadcrumbs and fried to a crunchy golden brown.

Makes 8 ● PREP TIME: 20 MINUTES

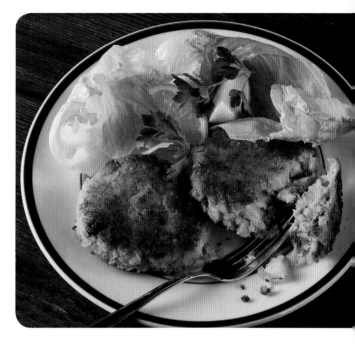

2 slices dry whole wheat bread

½ cup milk

2 cans (4 ounces each) fresh crabmeat

½ pound cooked shrimp, peeled, deveined, and chopped

2 large eggs, separated

2 teaspoons Dijon mustard

1 tablespoon Worcestershire sauce

½ cup ground almonds

Pinch of cayenne pepper

1 tablespoon mayonnaise

Handful of fresh parsley, rinsed, dried, and chopped

1½ cups dried low-sodium breadcrumbs

⅓ cup all-purpose flour

1 tablespoon water

Sunflower or canola oil

1 In a small bowl, soak bread in milk for 5 minutes.

2 Meanwhile, pick over crab to remove any cartilage. Into a medium bowl, flake the crabmeat and add shrimp. Add egg yolks, mustard, Worcestershire sauce, almonds, cayenne, and mayonnaise; then add 1 tablespoon parsley.

3 Squeeze bread dry, add it to crab and stir until soft but not sloppy. Add some dried breadcrumbs if mixture is too moist.

4 Put flour onto one plate and breadcrumbs onto another. In a shallow bowl, whisk water into egg whites.

5 Divide crab mixture into 8 portions and shape into cakes. Dip them into flour, and shake off excess; then dip them into egg whites and coat with breadcrumbs.

6 In a skillet over fairly high heat, heat ½ inch (1.5 cm) oil. Fry cakes until crisp and golden, 2 to 3 minutes on each side. Drain on a paper towel–lined plate and serve.

Per serving (2 cakes): 402 calories, 14 g total fat (2 g saturated), 32 g carbohydrates, 34 g protein, 3 g fiber, 255 mg cholesterol, 614 mg sodium, 195 mg calcium

Cajun Shrimp and Crab Jambalaya

This recipe brings home many favorites from the bayou, from shrimp and crab to the roux that flavors it all. We've substituted Canadian bacon for the high-fat chorizo sausage traditionally used in jambalaya. Cook up a double recipe for friends and serve it straight from the skillet, the down-home way.

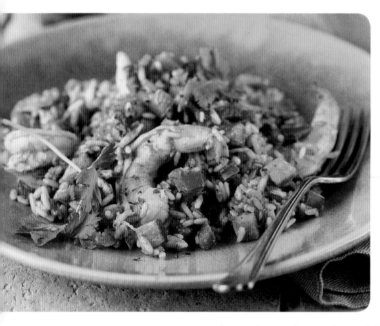

SERVES 6 • PREP TIME: 45 minutes

1 tablespoon vegetable oil

2 tablespoons all-purpose flour

2 medium onions, chopped

1 large green bell pepper, chopped

1 celery rib, chopped

3 ounces Canadian bacon, diced

1 can (28 ounces) chopped tomatoes in puree

1 can (14 ounces) reduced-sodium chicken broth

1½ cups long-grain white rice

2 teaspoons Old Bay seasoning

1 pound large shrimp, peeled and deveined

8 ounces lump crabmeat, picked through

2 tablespoons chopped fresh cilantro

1 Lightly coat a large, heavy skillet (preferably cast iron) with cooking spray and set over medium heat. Add oil and flour and stir constantly until roux turns a deep mahogany brown, about 5 minutes. Add onions, green pepper, celery, and bacon; sauté until vegetables are soft, about 5 minutes longer.

2 Stir in tomato, broth, rice, and Old Bay seasoning; bring to a boil over high heat. Reduce heat to medium-low, cover, and simmer until most of liquid is absorbed and rice is almost tender, about 20 minutes. Fold in shrimp and cook just until shrimp are pink and firm, about 5 minutes.

3 Gently fold in crab; cover and cook 1 minute. Remove from heat and let stand 3 minutes. Sprinkle with cilantro.

Per serving: 363 calories, 6 g total fat (1 g saturated), 45 g carbohydrates, 30 g protein, 2 g fiber, 152 mg cholesterol, 687 mg sodium

Salmon As You Like It

This recipe is just as easygoing as it sounds. Mix up any of these sweet, spicy, or savory marinades at right to make your omega 3–rich salmon a different dish every time.

Serves 1 ● PREP TIME: 20 minutes (plus up to 8 hours for marinating)

1 6-ounce center-cut salmon fillet

Olive oil

Whole wheat couscous

1½ cups mixed salad greens

Red, white, or sherry vinegar

Coarse salt and fresh-ground pepper to taste

1 Marinate salmon for a minimum of 15 minutes and a maximum of 8 hours in any of the marinade combinations below. (In a medium bowl, combine marinade ingredients, transfer to a large zipper-seal plastic bag, add salmon, seal tightly, and refrigerate.)

2 Prepare couscous as directed on package.

3 Meanwhile, heat grill to medium-high. Brush grill with olive oil; then cook salmon round side down for about 4 minutes. Turn and grill the other side until cooked through, 2 to 3 minutes.

4 Toss mixed salad greens with a swirl of olive oil, a dash of your favorite vinegar, and a pinch of salt and pepper.

Per serving (without marinade; includes couscous and salad with dressing): 504 calories, 30 g fat (5 g saturated), 25 g carbohydrates, 34 g protein, 5 g fiber, 85 mg cholesterol, 254 mg sodium

Prepared with Asian Blend: 549 calories, 33 g fat (5 g saturated), 29 g carbohydrates, 35 g protein, 5 g fiber, 85 mg cholesterol, 440 mg sodium

Prepared with Chimichurri Blend: 517 calories, 31 g fat (5 g saturated), 25 g carbohydrates, 34 g protein, 5 g fiber, 85 mg cholesterol, 255 mg sodium

Prepared with Tex-Mex Blend: 510 calories, 30 g fat (5 g saturated), 26 g carbohydrates, 34 g protein, 6 g fiber, 85 mg cholesterol, 389 mg sodium

NOTE:
Nutritional analyses with marinades are for 1 serving and include salmon, couscous, and salad with dressing. Marinades were calculated with a 10–15% absorption rate, since much of the marinade gets discarded.

Asian Blend

2 tablespoons olive oil

1 teaspoon sesame oil

2 tablespoons soy sauce

2 tablespoons balsamic vinegar

1 tablespoon honey or agave syrup

1½ teaspoons brown sugar

½ teaspoon ground ginger

A pinch of crushed red pepper flakes

1 large shallot, finely chopped

1 clove garlic, finely chopped

Juice of ½ lime or lemon

Chimichurri Blend

1 tablespoon lemon juice

1 tablespoon olive oil

1½ tablespoons finely chopped scallion

1½ tablespoons minced fresh parsley

1 garlic clove, smashed and finely chopped

Pinch of pepper

Pinch of crushed red pepper flakes or cayenne pepper

Tex-Mex Blend

¼ cup tomato sauce or ketchup

1 can (4 ounces) chopped green chilies

1 tablespoon fresh lime juice

1 teaspoon chili powder

1 teaspoon ground cumin

¼ teaspoon salt

¼ teaspoon pepper

Dash of hot pepper sauce

Fish Tacos

Next to salmon and mackerel, halibut is one of the richest sources of omega-3 fatty acids you can put on your plate. These tangy fish tacos put this sweet-flavored white fish front and center.

MAKES 8 ● PREP TIME: 30 Minutes

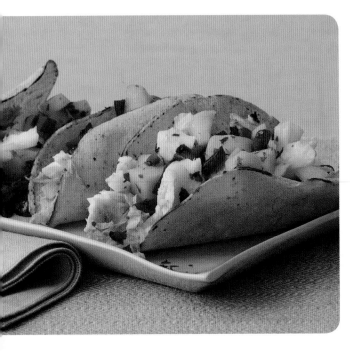

1 tablespoon olive oil

2 cloves garlic, minced

1 teaspoon ground cumin

½ teaspoon salt

3 tablespoons lime juice

1½ pounds halibut fillets

1 ripe mango, peeled, seeded, and chopped

½ small red bell pepper, seeded and finely chopped

½ jalapeño pepper, seeded, deveined, and finely chopped (wear gloves when handling; they burn)

¼ cup chopped cilantro (optional)

8 soft corn tortillas (8-inch/20-cm)

1 cup shredded lettuce

1 Preheat broiler. Coat a broiler pan with cooking spray. In a medium bowl, combine oil, garlic, cumin, salt, 1 tablespoon lime juice, and fish; toss to coat. Let stand 15 minutes.

2 In a small bowl, combine mango, bell pepper, jalapeño, cilantro, if desired, and remaining 2 tablespoons lime juice. Set aside.

3 Wrap tortillas in foil. Remove fish from marinade and place on broiler pan. Broil until opaque, 3 to 6 minutes. Transfer to a plate and place tortillas in oven to warm slightly, about 1 minute. Flake the fish.

4 Top tortillas with equal amounts of lettuce, fish, and salsa.

Per serving (2 tacos): 380 calories, 9 g total fat (2 g saturated), 36 g carbohydrates, 39 g protein, 5 g fiber, 54 mg cholesterol, 430 mg sodium

Lentil and Bean Chili

Nothing takes the chill out of a fall evening like a bowl of steaming, spicy chili. Lentils and beans team up in this hearty vegetarian version that is rich in soluble fiber and protein, both strong weight-loss allies. Garnish with diced avocado, chopped fresh cilantro and scallions, and grated pepper Jack or cheddar cheese.

SERVES 8 • Prep time: 1 hour

2 teaspoons olive oil

1 cup chopped onion (1 medium)

1 cup diced carrots (2–4 medium)

3 cloves garlic, minced

5 teaspoons chili powder

4 teaspoons ground cumin

1 teaspoon dried oregano

4 cups vegetable broth or reduced-sodium chicken broth

¾ cup brown lentils, sorted and rinsed

2 cans (10 ounces) diced tomatoes with green chiles

2 cans (15 or 19 ounces each) dark red kidney beans, drained and rinsed

Freshly ground pepper to taste

1 In a Dutch oven, heat oil over medium heat. Add onion and carrots. Cook, stirring often, until softened, 3 to 5 minutes.

2 Add garlic, chili powder, cumin, and oregano. Cook, stirring, until fragrant, 30 to 60 seconds. Add broth and lentils. Bring to a simmer. Reduce heat to medium-low, cover, and simmer for 25 minutes.

3 Add tomatoes, kidney beans, and pepper. Return to a simmer. Cook, covered, over medium-low heat until lentils are tender, 15 to 20 minutes longer.

Per serving *(1 cup):* 199 calories, 3 g total fat, (0 g saturated), 36 g carbohydrates, 12 g protein, 12 g fiber, 0 mg cholesterol, 691 mg sodium

Veggie Tacos
with Homemade Salsa and Guacamole

This colorful and filling main course is low in saturated fat but high in flavor.

MAKES 8 • PREP TIME: 45 minutes

2 tablespoons extra-virgin olive oil

1 onion, finely chopped

1 eggplant (10 ounces), cubed

1 butternut squash (1½ pounds), halved, seeded, peeled, and cubed

1 large zucchini (6 ounces), cubed

¼ teaspoon chili powder

½ teaspoon ground cumin

1 garlic clove, crushed

1 can (14½ ounces) tomatoes

Salt and pepper, to taste

1 large ripe avocado

Juice of ½ lime

3 ripe tomatoes, diced

½ red onion, finely chopped

¼ cup chopped cilantro

8 taco shells

8 ounces plain low-fat yogurt

Lime wedges and fresh cilantro for garnish

1 In large saucepan, heat oil over medium-high heat. Add white onion and eggplant and sauté, stirring frequently, until vegetables are lightly browned.

2 Add squash and zucchini. Stir in chili powder, cumin, and garlic. Pour in canned tomatoes with juice. Add salt and pepper to taste. Heat to boiling, breaking up tomatoes with wooden spoon. Cover and simmer 15 minutes, stirring occasionally, until squash is just tender. During cooking, add water if needed, to prevent vegetables from sticking.

3 Meanwhile, preheat oven to 350°F (177°C). To make guacamole, halve and pit avocado, scoop out flesh into a bowl, and mash with lime juice. To make salsa, in a separate bowl, mix together fresh tomatoes, red onion, and cilantro. Set guacamole and salsa aside.

4 Put taco shells on baking sheet and warm in oven for 3 to 4 minutes. Transfer shells to serving plates. Fill with eggplant mixture. Top with guacamole, yogurt, and salsa. Garnish with lime wedges and cilantro and serve.

Per serving: (*2 tacos*): 420 calories, 21 g total fat (3 g saturated), 56 g carbohydrates, 8 g protein, 15 g fiber, 0 mg cholesterol, 150 mg sodium

Penne with Fresh Tomato Sauce and Grilled Zucchini

If you like pasta, this dish will become one of your weeknight standbys. It's simple, fresh, light, and there's a minimum of cooking involved.

SERVES 4 ● PREP TIME: 20 minutes

3 medium ripe tomatoes, cored and cut into ½-inch (1.5-cm) chunks

2 tablespoons balsamic vinegar

3 tablespoons extra-virgin olive oil

1 teaspoon salt

½ teaspoon ground black pepper

12 ounces penne, preferably whole-grain

4 medium zucchini, rinsed and ends trimmed

¼ cup minced fresh oregano or basil

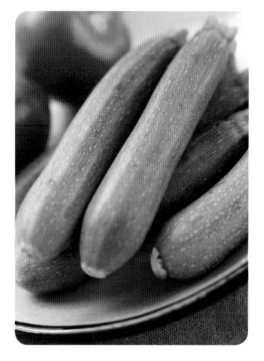

1 In a bowl large enough to hold the pasta, add tomato chunks. Stir in vinegar, oil, ½ teaspoon salt, and ¼ teaspoon pepper. Set aside.

2 Heat grill to medium-high.

3 In a large pot of boiling salted water, cook pasta until just tender, 8 to 10 minutes.

4 Meanwhile, cut zucchini lengthwise into slabs about ½ inch (1.5 cm) thick. Transfer to a baking sheet coated with cooking spray. Sprinkle with remaining ½ teaspoon salt and ¼ teaspoon pepper.

5 Grill zucchini until nicely grill-marked but not limp, about 4 minutes per side.

6 Transfer to a cutting board and chop into ½-inch (1.5-cm) chunks. Add to bowl with tomatoes.

7 Drain pasta and add to the bowl, along with the oregano or basil. Stir gently to mix. Serve hot or warm.

Per serving: 464 calories, 13 g total fat (1 g saturated), 73 g carbohydrates, 15 g protein, 6 g fiber, 612 mg sodium

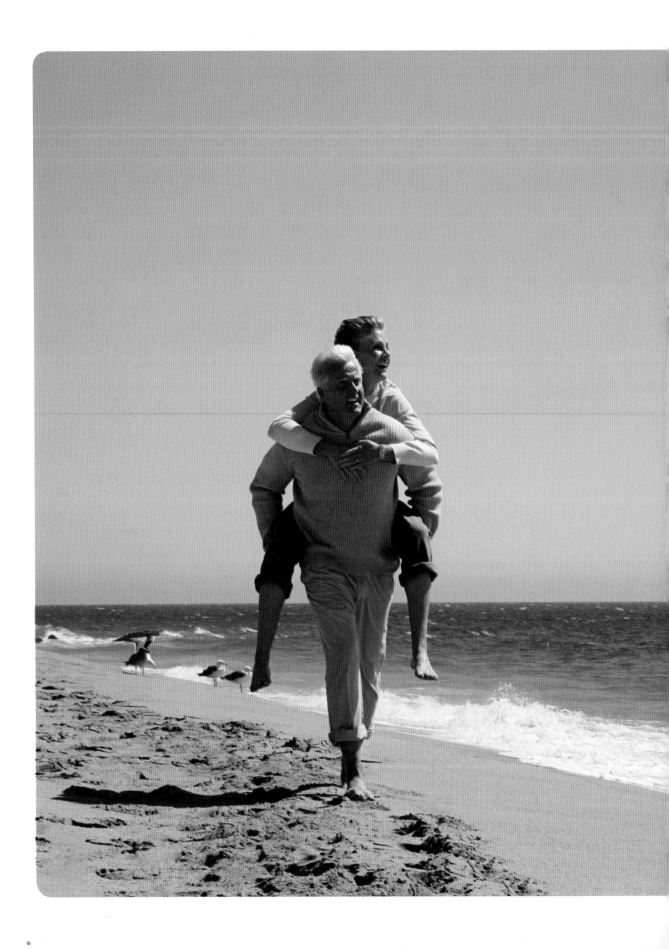

More Places
to Walk

WALKING AS A LIFESTYLE is more than just lacing up your sneakers and hitting the street once a day. It's about looking for opportunities to walk whenever possible and getting genuine pleasure out of your efforts—whatever the season, whatever the reason, wherever you are. You'll know you're a real walker when you find yourself thinking, I bet that would be a great place to walk. This chapter is full of ways and places to get you walking outside your comfort zone.

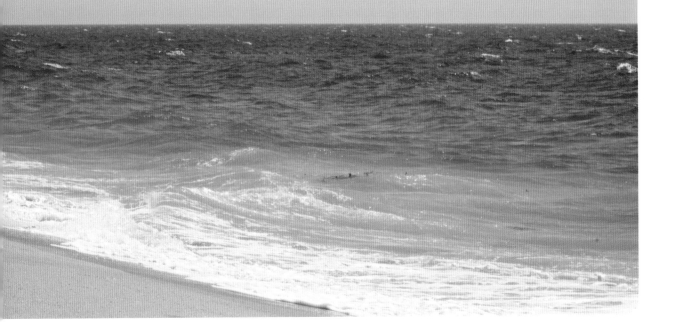

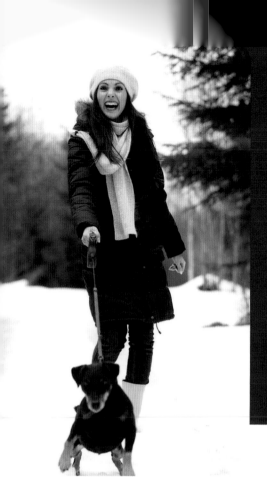

For *Every Season* There's a Reason

It's not just your morning walk or your Sunday stroll anymore. It's also your spring or fall hike, your summer beachcombing, and your winter trek. Each provides a different added pleasure and challenge to your ordinary walks. Weather and climate, as well as terrain, provide the seasonal change-ups that can make walking an adventure (see " 'Weather' to Walk" on page 33). And each season gives you a new reason to get out there and do what comes naturally.

Hike the Natural Beauty of Spring and Fall

When spring has sprung or autumn foliage calls, head for the hills. Whether your pleasure is plunging waterfalls, stark walls of granite, flowering meadows, or groves of giant trees, chances are that within a fairly easy drive of where you live, there's a park where you can walk among such natural beauty. However, in these settings it's not walking; it's hiking! If you've been walking for fitness, then getting off the proverbial beaten path—or sidewalk—will bring a whole new level of excitement, along with lots of soul-satisfying views, to your routine.

Here are some ways to ensure your trek is both enjoyable and safe.

Research the trails. Planning a hike is half the fun, and there's certainly no shortage of worthy destinations. In the national park system alone, there are 17,000 miles of trails in 49 states, says Jamie Patten, a spokesperson for the National Park Foundation. (Only Delaware doesn't have a national park of its own.) And every state has more than a dozen state parks, with hundreds of thousands of miles of trails between them. You can scour local guidebooks for recommendations or go to www.nps.gov or www.stateparks.com and click on your state for information about specific parks. "If the woods aren't your thing, lots of urban, military, and historic parks have trails that lead you through magnificent gardens," says Patten.

Once you've chosen a destination, you'll need to choose a trail, and choose it wisely. "If you're new to hiking, it's better to begin with hikes that are described as easy or moderate," advises Emily Williams, director of programs for the Tahoe Rim Trail Association in Incline Village, Nevada. Consider the length of the hike—3 to 5 miles (5 to 8 km) is a good place to start if you're fairly fit—the altitude, and elevation changes. A 5-mile hike in a park that's at 3,000 feet (914 m) elevation and involves 2,000 feet (610 m) of climbing will be a very different experience than the same distance on a flat trail at sea level. When in doubt, choose a shorter hike than you think you can do. You can always do a longer trail next time.

Bring along a Detailed Trail Map and GPS. Many park websites provide trail maps, but some aren't very detailed and could leave you scratching your head at a fork in the trail. Do yourself a favor and stop in the park office before your hike and buy a better map. If you're using a map from a guidebook, make a copy of the map to keep in your backpack so you don't have to carry the whole book.

Global Positioning System (GPS) units all use the same system of satellites—originally developed for the military—as reference points that calculate where the GPS unit is on the ground. To mark your starting position, all you have to do is turn the unit on. From there you mark locations along the route, called waypoints, that act as digital breadcrumbs to help you find your way back using the same route. The GPS will also tell you which direction you need to go if you get off track. (Never rely solely on a GPS; you should always carry a trail map and compass as backups and mark your coordinates on the map before you depart.) Be sure to practice using your GPS before you take it into the wilderness.

Dress Smartly. There's a saying about mountain weather: If you want it to change, wait five minutes. You can set out in nothing but sunshine and midway through the

LOSE YOURSELF

It's time to get lost in one of these fragrant forests, designated fall's best by www.gorp.away.com.

- Willamette National Forest, OR
- Inyo National Forest, CA
- Coconino National Forest, AZ
- Gunnison National Forest, CO
- Chequamegon-Nicolet National Forest, WI
- Mark Twain National Forest, MO
- Pisgah National Forest, NC
- Allegheny National Forest, PA
- Green Mountain National Forest, VT
- White Mountain National Forest, NH-ME

PUT SOME SPRING IN YOUR STEP

Get outside! There's nothing like a warm breeze and the gentle light of spring to get your vitamin D levels where they ought to be and boost your mood.

Be social. Spring is about new beginnings; it's also a wonderful time to renew old friendships. Invite someone on a walk today.

Get fit to go sleeveless. No doubt you'll be sporting more warm-weather clothes. Try using walking poles to tone your upper body.

Go somewhere pretty. A British study found that a 30-minute walk in a country park lowered depression far more than an indoor jaunt of the same length.

hike be caught in a sudden rain shower. The best advice is simply to wear layers. That way, you'll be prepared for a range of temperatures (remember, the higher you hike, the colder it will get).

Of course, you can hike in jeans or shorts, a T-shirt, and sturdy athletic shoes, but clothing made from quick-drying technical fabrics will be more comfortable. We suggest a shirt made of a lightweight synthetic fabric, a warm mid-layer top made from a fabric such as fleece, and a lightweight rain shell. You'll should also bring a hat or visor and some sunblock.

As for your feet, whether you wear traditional above-the-ankle hiking boots or a sturdy pair of shoes depends on the terrain you plan to tackle. On rocky terrain you'll want a boot with hefty soles that will protect your feet from "stone bruises" and provide enough support and stability to keep you from twisting an ankle. On smoother terrain you can wear shoes that resemble running shoes but have extra traction.

Keep safety in mind. For safety's sake, it's a good idea to carry a few key items, including a small flashlight with fresh batteries, a compass or GPS, and a first-aid kit containing bandages, tweezers (to remove splinters), and antihistamine tablets (for bee stings). Also bring a whistle. If you get injured or lost, blow three times—that's the signal for "I need help." As for snacks, bring foods that pack a lot of energy into a small space, such as nuts, protein bars, peanut butter sandwiches, and beef jerky (see "Top 20 Power Foods for Walkers," page 122).

Practice good trail etiquette. If you're hiking with a group of friends, and another hiker or a smaller group approaches, step aside and let the lone hiker or smaller group pass. For safety, hikers should yield to anyone on horseback. And always abide by the "Leave no trace" principles, which include respecting wildlife, staying on durable paths rather than tramping on vulnerable land, and the most obvious: putting trash where it belongs, even if that means you have to carry it for miles.

Pace yourself. If you're hiking with a group, let the least fit person—even if it's a child—set the pace. Remember, you don't just have to reach the vista the trail leads to; you also have to get back!

MAKE YOUR OWN HIKING SNACKS

Tote-Along Bagel Chips
Preheat oven to 425°F (218°C). Slice one whole wheat bagel horizontally into 4 slices. Then cut each of the slices into 6 pieces. Spread the bagel pieces onto a large baking sheet and spray them with olive-oil cooking spray. In a small bowl combine 2 tablespoons grated Parmesan cheese, 1 tablespoon dried basil, 2 teaspoons dried oregano, 2 teaspoons garlic powder, 1 teaspoon onion powder, and salt and pepper to taste. Sprinkle the chips with this herb mixture.

Bake for about 5 to 6 minutes until lightly toasted. Store in a zipper-seal bag.

Perfectly Roasted Pumpkin Seeds
Separate the seeds from the pumpkin flesh, wash well, and let dry. Then place in a bowl and mix with a small amount of canola oil and salt. Spread in one layer on a baking sheet and sprinkle on some cinnamon, paprika, or chili powder if you like. Bake at 300F (149°C) for about 45 minutes, shaking and stirring occasionally.

WHAT TO WEAR IN THE WOODS

Take a hike? Sure, why not! You might get away with wearing just your gym shorts and a tee, plus good-quality hiking or walking shoes. But soon you'll be wondering how it got so hot (or so cold) outside or how you got so thirsty (or hungry). Here's the gear you don't want to hike without:

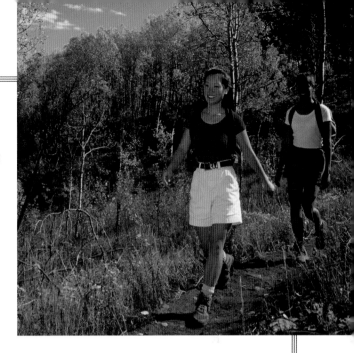

Sunglasses

Look for impact-resistant polarized lenses that provide 100 percent protection from harmful UV rays. High SPF sunblock is a good idea, too.

Trail shorts or pants

These should be made of a fast-drying synthetic fabric with a touch of spandex for comfort. A lined waistband will wick away sweat, while vents at the hems let you breathe. Wear pants banded at the ankle to keep woodland ticks at bay

Layering tees and jackets

Depending on the temperature, you'll want to wear a short- or long-sleeved T-shirt in a light fabric that wicks away sweat to keep you dry and comfortable, and a light quick-drying and breathable jacket. A hood is nice in the event of an unexpected shower or a chill.

Hiking shoes and socks

Hiking shoes or boots with breathable waterproof material and toe protection provide comfort and safety, whatever the weather. And socks made of quick-drying, wick-away fabric make a big difference, too.

Walking poles

Walking with poles increases the number of calories you burn by about 20 percent, reduces stress on your joints, and encourages good walking posture. Plus, on rocky terrain or steep hills poles provide added stability.

Water bottle

Get yourself one of those handy, sturdy BPA-free bottles designed to hook to your waist or backpack.

Snacks

Hikers rely on trail mix because it keeps well, provides plenty of protein and energy, and doesn't take up much room. Start with nuts and raisins and add any of these: dried apples, cranberries, cherries, or bananas; pumpkin or sunflower seeds; roasted soybeans (also called soy nuts); granola; or breakfast cereal.

Carry enough water. A classic beginner hiker's mistake is to set out without enough water. Yes, water is heavy, so when you're choosing a trail, make sure it's short enough that you can walk it with a little extra weight. Plan to carry about 1 quart of liquid per person for every two hours of hiking. A word to the wise: Never drink from streams. Even if the water looks pristine, it is likely filled with bacteria or other organisms that can make you very sick.

Savor Summer

Ah, summer! Here comes the sun—and if you're lucky, a long-awaited trip to the beach. Walking the sandy shores is one of the best workouts around. For one, packed sand is firm but far more forgiving on your joints than a cement sidewalk. Because it is soft enough to have some "give," however, it forces you to work a little harder and use more energy—hence, burn more calories. In fact, walking in sand burns about 50 percent more calories than trucking along at the same pace on a more solid surface.

The beach is a unique walking surface that requires some special attention. Here are some tips for successful walks on the sand.

Find the flat stretches. The shoreline naturally falls toward the ocean at an angle. Over time this can be hard on your ankles, knees, and hips. Try to find the flattest surface possible. If there is none, alter the direction you walk daily to create more even stress on your body.

Wear shoes. Bare feet are fine for short jaunts and playing around. But walking longer stretches on the sand in bare feet stresses your lower leg muscles and connective tissues and can lead to shin splints and sore Achilles tendons. If you're going to walk any longer than a few minutes, do so in shoes, such as light sneakers or supportive sandals.

Break it up. Beach walking can be tiring because it takes more energy than you're used to putting out during your regular walking workouts. Break it up with the toning exercises (see "Beach Ball Moves" on page 194) to use your muscles in a different way and give your body a break.

Shape Up at the Shore

The following three 30-minute workouts mix walking with toning exercises and will keep you in swimsuit shape despite those evening ice-cream runs. Simply rotate through them, taking one day in between for a long, leisurely walk at your own pace. Finally, the "Beach Ball Moves" on page 194 will help you shape up without ever leaving your beach blanket.

HOOKED ON HIKING? TRY AN OVERNIGHTER

Once you get hooked on hiking, you might want to take it to the next level and try an overnight trip. With a little bit of digging, you can find outfitters that offer hut-to-hut trips or overnight trips with "van" support, meaning you hike but don't have to carry your gear. Here are a few.

In the East The Appalachian Mountain Club (www.outdoors.org) offers short guided trips in the White Mountains.

In the Rockies Aspen Alpine Guides (www.aspenalpine.com) offers trips in which hikers can carry their own packs or opt for van support.

In the West The Sierra Club owns half a dozen huts in the Sierra Nevada range (no guided trips). Hikers reserve space in the huts before they set out (www.sierraclub.org).

In Europe Slow Travel (www.slowtrav.com) offers guided hut-to-hut trips throughout Europe.

BEACH WORKOUT #1

Lower-Body Blast

Firm up those stubbornly soft bikini-bottom muscles with this great lower-body, fat-blasting, muscle-toning workout. All you need is a pair of walking shoes and a stretch of sand.

5 minutes	**Warm up** Start by strolling, gradually picking up your pace until you're moving briskly and breathing harder, but not out of breath. Remember to bend your arms and propel yourself by pumping your arms more quickly. Your feet will naturally follow.
5 minutes	**Brisk walking**
2 minutes	**Lunge series (page 188)** Do 10 to 12 walking lunges, followed by 10 to 12 lateral lunges, followed by 10 to 12 back lunges.
2 minutes	**Walk at an easy pace**
10 minutes	**Brisk walking**
2 minutes	**Squat series (page 189)** Do 10 to 15 high-hand squats, then 10 to 16 side-kick squats.
4 minutes	**Cool down** Walk at an easy pace to stretch your legs and cool down.

SUMMER STRATEGIES

Sleep with the shades up. The sun will help you rise and shine in time for a cool morning walk.

Hit the farmer's market. Bring a big bag; you won't go home empty-handed.

Light up the grill. Turn off the stove and take the cooking outside.

Walk the beach. Soft sand provides the best exercise around.

Turn off the tube. People who watch less TV weigh less. And summer's too short to waste.

Forward Lunge

Stand with your feet hip-width apart, hands on hips. Take a giant step forward with your right foot, plant it on the ground, and bend both knees, lowering straight down toward the ground. Press into your right foot, straightening both legs, and immediately lunge forward with the left leg. Continue alternating for the full set.

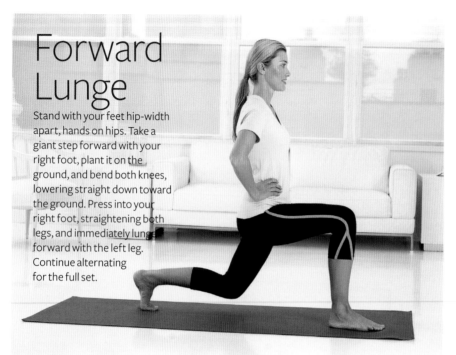

Back Lunge

Stand with your feet hip-width apart, hands on hips. Take a giant step back with your right leg. Immediately bend your left leg and slowly lower your right knee toward the ground. Press into your left foot, and straighten both legs to return to the starting position. Repeat with the opposite leg. Continue alternating for a full set.

Lateral Lunge

Stand with your feet together, arms at your sides. Take a giant step to the left. As you plant your left foot, bend your left knee and lower your butt toward the ground until your left thigh is nearly parallel to the floor. Do not allow your left knee to jut past your toes. Bend forward and touch the floor with the fingertips of both hands. Then push back up to the starting position. Repeat to the other side. Alternate for a full set.

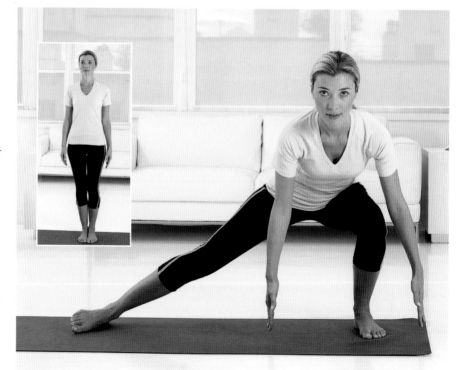

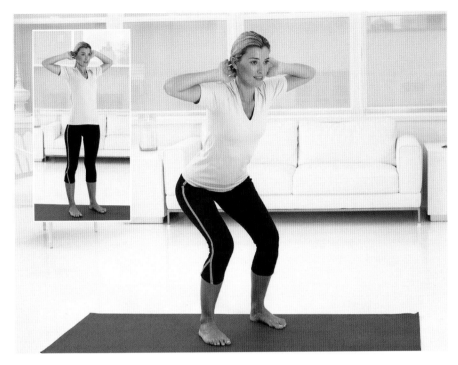

High-Hand Squats

Stand with your feet slightly wider than shoulder-width apart, hands behind your head. Keeping your elbows wide, bend your knees and extend your butt behind you as if you're about to sit; your legs should be bent close to 90 degrees and your thighs nearly parallel to the ground. Press back up to the starting position and repeat.

Side-Kick Squats

Stand with your feet close together, hands on your hips. Bend your knees and extend your butt behind you until your legs are bent about 45 degrees in a partial squat. Press back up to the starting position. Once standing, immediately raise your left leg out to the side as far as comfortably possible. Lower back to start. Perform another squat and repeat the leg lift to the opposite side. Continue alternating for a full set.

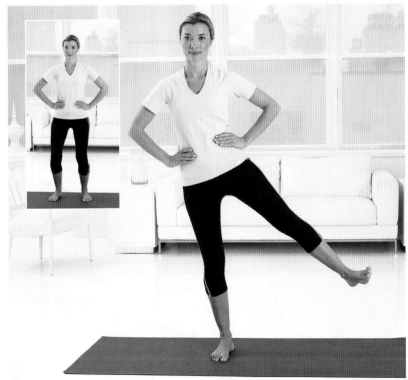

BEACH WORKOUT #2

Cardio Core Sculpt & Stroll

This workout tightens and tones your core muscles while keeping your heart rate in a fat-burning zone. You might want to carry a light towel for this workout (one that you can easily sling around the back of your neck), since you'll be lying down in the sand.

5 minutes	**Warm up** Start by strolling, gradually picking up your pace until you're moving briskly and breathing harder, but not out of breath. Remember to bend your arms and propel yourself by pumping your arms more quickly. Your feet will naturally follow.
5 minutes	**Brisk walking**
2 minutes	**Curl Down, Curl Up (page 192)** Do 2 sets of 8 to 10 reps, with 30 seconds' rest between sets.
5 minutes	**Brisk walking**
2 minutes	**Plank Twist (page 192)** Do 2 sets of 6 to 8 reps, with 30 to 60 seconds' rest between sets.
5 minutes	**Brisk walking**.
2 minutes	**Plank Glute Press (page 193)** Do 2 sets of 8 to 10 reps, with 30 seconds' rest between sets..
4 minutes	**Cool down** Walk at an easy pace to stretch your legs and cool down.

Double-Trouble Challenge

This workout takes advantage of the different terrain available on the beach. Walking in the soft sand requires more of a push off from your calves, hamstrings, and glutes, so it's great for challenging and firming those muscles as well as burning more calories. Switching to harder sand gives you a little break.

5 minutes	Start by strolling on the firm sand, gradually picking up your pace until you're moving briskly and you're breathing harder but aren't out of breath. Remember to bend your arms and propel yourself by pumping your arms more quickly. Your feet will naturally follow..
5 minutes	Move onto the soft sand. Try to maintain the same general effort as when you were walking on the firm sand, though your pace may slow down. Concentrate on taking powerful strides and maintaining good form.
3 minutes	Recover with brisk walking on the firm sand.
5 minutes	Move onto the soft sand. Try to maintain the same general effort as when you were walking on the firm sand, though your pace may slow down. Concentrate on taking powerful strides and maintaining good form.
4 minutes	Move to the soft sand and walk as quickly as you can, maintaining good form.
8 minutes	Recover with brisk walking on the firm sand, taking the last two to three minutes at an easy pace to cool down.

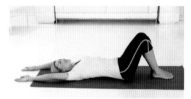

Curl Down, Curl Up

Sit with legs bent, feet flat on the ground, and arms extended at chest height. Lift your breastbone to sit tall. Contracting your abs for control, slowly roll down one vertebra at a time, allowing your spine to curve naturally and your arms to come overhead as you lie back onto the ground. Slowly curl back up.

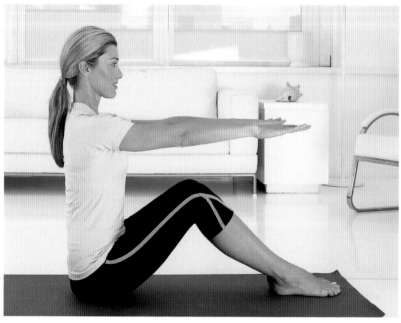

Plank Twist

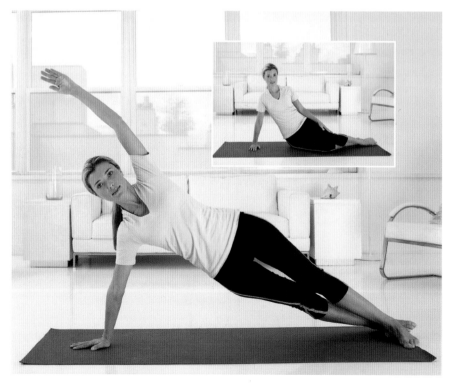

Sit on your right hip with your legs to the side and your left foot just in front of the right. Place your right hand on the ground beneath your right shoulder, and your left hand on your left leg. In one motion contract your obliques (side torso muscles), lift your hips off the ground, and sweep your left arm overhead so that your body forms a diagonal line. Hold for two breaths, then slowly lower and repeat.

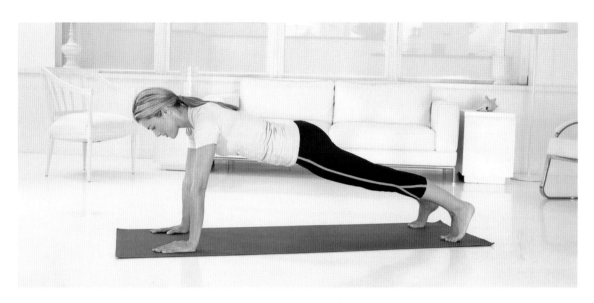

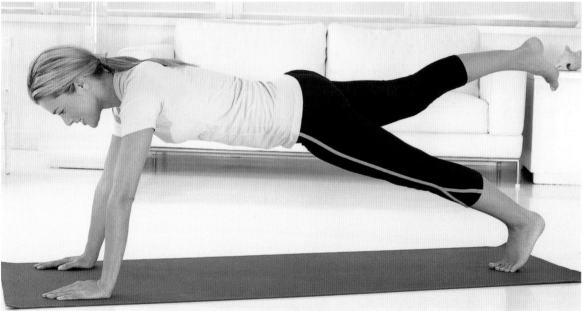

Plank Glute Press

Assume a push-up position with your hands directly beneath your shoulders and your legs extended straight behind you, balancing on your toes. Keeping your abs tight and your back straight, contract your glutes and raise your right leg off the ground as far as comfortably possible. Hold for two breaths. Then lower and repeat for a full set before switching sides and performing the move with the left leg.

Beach Ball Moves

Grab a beach ball and firm up with these easy exercises you can do at home or right on your beach blanket. Do 2 sets of 10 to 15 reps of each move.

▶ Ball Hug

Hold a large, firm beach ball between your hands, elbows pointing out to the sides. Contract your chest muscles and squeeze the ball as firmly as possible for a count of 4. Release the ball slightly, then squeeze again. Tones chest and shoulders.

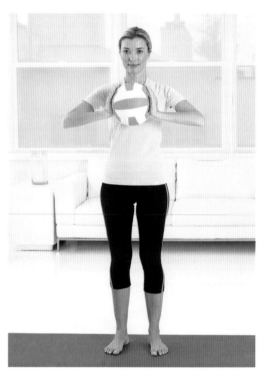

▼ Beach Ball Squeeze

Lie on your back with arms at your sides. Place a large, firm beach ball between your knees and shins and raise your legs until your thighs are perpendicular to the ground. Keep your feet flexed. Using your inner thigh muscles, slowly squeeze the ball for a count of 4. Pause, then slowly release the ball to a count of 4 without completely releasing tension. Tones inner thighs.

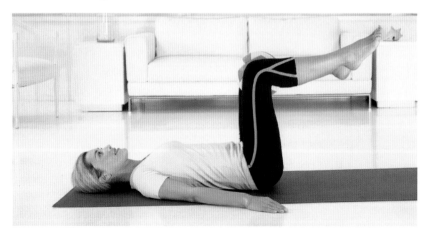

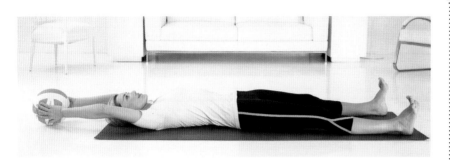

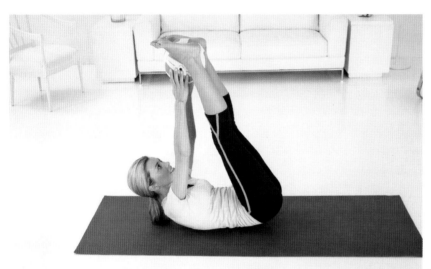

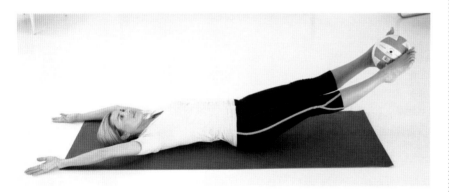

▲ Hands to Feet

Lie back with your legs extended, feet flexed. Hold the beach ball with both hands and extend your arms back over your head. Keeping your arms and legs extended, elbows and knees soft, contract your abs and raise your arms and legs toward each other. When your hands and feet are directly over your body, switch the ball from your hands to your feet, then immediately lower your arms and legs back to the starting position. Repeat, this time switching the ball from your feet to your hands. That's 1 rep. Repeat for a full set. Tones core.

Winter Walkabout

Winter often gets a bad rap. It has been said that it was invented so we'll appreciate the rest of the seasons. And unless you're a snow- and cold-loving skier or ice skater, the temptation to hunker down and hibernate for the winter is very real. If you do that, though, you might miss some of the prettiest, most invigorating walks of the whole year! Nothing's lovelier than a walk in the quiet after snowfall, after all. You don't need to punish yourself, walking in icy conditions or through a blizzard, for heaven's sake. Just learn how to dress smart for winter walking and make up your mind to get out there on the clear days.

Dress in layers.

Wear layers of breathable fabrics that draw moisture away from the body and dry quickly. Start with a thin base layer, followed by a thermal layer, then an outer shell that breaks the wind and cold. Fabrics such as Thinsulate, Gortex, Thermax, fleece, and wool are good choices. Avoid cotton, though, because it holds on to moisture.

Cover your head and hands.

Your mom was right about keeping your head warm in winter. Wear a hat, preferably one with earflaps if you're one of those people with perpetually cold ears. A scarf or cowl keeps the cold from sneaking in at the neck. On your hands, weatherproof mittens are your best bet.

Take care of your feet.

You can peel off or add on layers of clothing as you walk in winter, but you're pretty much stuck with what you've got on your feet. And nothing's more important. If your walking surface is dry and clear, your regular walking shoes are fine. Otherwise, waterproof hiking boots are best for keeping your feet warm and dry and providing traction for safety. Wear fabric-appropriate socks (see pages 31–32 for more info on socks), with one thin layer under another if necessary. Winter walking rule of thumb: If your feet get wet, go home. Carrying a spare pair of socks won't hurt, but it's best to get your feet warm and dry as quickly as possible.

WHAT ABOUT SNOWSHOES?

Walking in snowshoes is fun, not to mention great exercise; you burn about 40 percent more calories when snowshoeing than regular walking at the same speed. The only gear you need besides your ordinary winter wear are those snowshoes, which will set you back between $100 and $200 for a good beginner pair. Trekking or ski poles can help you maintain your balance and navigate terrain, but they're not a must.

WINTER HEALTH GUIDE

You're already fighting colds by walking nearly every day—studies prove it. Researchers from the University of South Carolina found that adults who exercised moderately to vigorously at least four times a week had 25 percent fewer colds over one year than those who moved less. So one of the best ways to prevent winter colds is to keep walking! Here are a few other strategies that can help lower your risk for catching cold that can keep you on your feet all winter long.

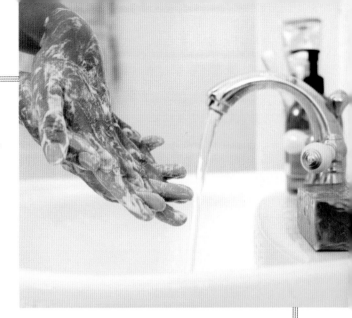

Hand washing

Nasty cold viruses can survive for up to seven days on light switches, ATMs, doorknobs, and other surfaces—and for at least three hours on unwashed hands. Scrub up to five times a day with soap and water, lathering vigorously for 20 seconds, rinsing thoroughly, then drying your hands with a clean paper towel. If you're using a public restroom, use the paper towel to turn off the faucet and to open the door when you leave.

Alcohol-based hand sanitizers

Use them when you can't get to a sink—they're not perfect, but they're much better than nothing. Look for a product that contains at least 70 percent ethanol alcohol, which is the minimum level of alcohol required to combat the rhinoviruses that cause colds. Don't let the gel build up on your hands after multiple uses. When you can get to a sink, wash up.

Saline nasal spray

Moist nasal passages are less receptive to cold viruses than dry ones. In one 20-week study, subjects who used a saline nasal spray every day had 30 percent fewer colds and 42 percent fewer days with runny noses or congestion. Spritz regularly in the winter, when heated indoor air is dry and during airplane flights.

Probiotics

A recent Austrian study showed that germ-eating white blood cells called macrophages became more active in women who consumed either a probiotic supplement or 3.5 to 7 ounces of yogurt a day for a month. "Good" bacteria commonly added to yogurt also increase levels of an important infection-fighting protein and rev up white blood cells called lymphocytes.

Sleep

Ever notice how when feeling you're tired, you're more likely to get sick? That's because getting enough shut-eye keeps your immune system strong and when you're sleep deprived and rundown, well, you're a winter cold waiting to happen. Sticking to a regular sleep schedule is key, as is not letting the TV or computer, as well as alcohol and coffee, from interfering with your sleep.

Flu fighters

A cold is annoying, but the flu can lay you flat out in the winter. To keep the flu at bay, get a flu shot or prescription nasal mist at the beginning of each flu season; these can provide from 40 to 90 percent protection against the strains of the flu that are common in any given year. The minute someone in your household exhibits flu symptoms, as your doctor for Tamiflu or Relenza for yourself; these antiviral drugs can significantly reduce your chance of catching the flu from your housemate. Finally, if you can drive or take a train instead of flying, do it. Nothing puts you at risk like air travel. Besides the people coughing and sneezing on you in airports and sitting next to you on the plane, the recirculated air and germy surfaces don't do you any favors either. If you must fly, take the first flight out in the morning because the plane will have been recently cleaned from the previous day. And don't forget your hand sanitizer!

HOME-BREWED CHAI

Combine 1½ cups water, ¼ teaspoon ground cinnamon, ¼ teaspoon ground cloves, and ¼ teaspoon ground ginger in a small saucepan. Bring to a low boil, reduce heat to low, cover, and simmer for 5 minutes. Add ⅔ cup 1% low-fat milk or vanilla soymilk and heat until steaming. Remove from the heat. Add three black tea bags, cover, and let steep for 3 to 4 minutes. Pour into two mugs and sweeten each with a spot of honey. Only 60 calories per serving!

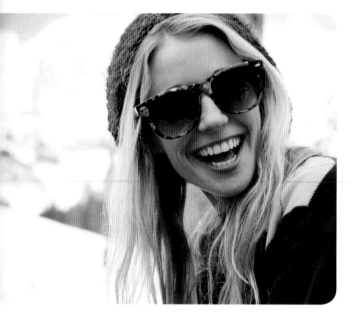

BE SURE TO USE HIGH SPF SUNSCREEN ON EXPOSED SKIN, EVEN IN WINTER.

Mind the sun.

Just because it's 20°F (–7°C) doesn't mean you can't get a sunburn. Wear sunglasses and sunblock, just as you would during the other seasons. And bring water along, too, because hydration is important every day of the year.

Watch where you're going.

Winter is not the time to get lost in a mad revelry of rap and R&B on your MP3 player. A patch of ice or a winter-damaged walking surface can sneak up on you suddenly, with the potential of turning your pleasant walk into a trip to the emergency room. Pay careful attention to what's ahead, giving yourself time and clearance to walk around or away from dicey conditions.

Consider the Wind.

Some people can handle the cold but just can't abide the wind. Maybe that's because of wind chill, where 10 m.p.h. winds make the temperature feel 15 degrees colder than it is, and for every additional 5 m.p.h. of wind, it feels another 5 degrees colder. Brrrr. Walk in the wind if you want to, but take the cold, hard facts of wind chill into account when you're dressing: Layers, layers, layers, and cover your head, face, neck, and hands.

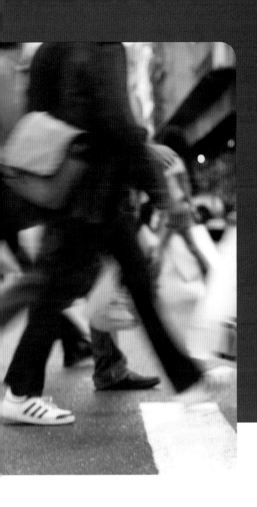

Experience *Vacations* on Foot

By now you know how to turn your Saturday errands or an afternoon at your kid's soccer field into a Walk It Off weight-loss opportunity. Whatever you're doing, walk while you're doing it. That's called living the walking lifestyle. But what about when you're not in your regular routine, say, when you're on vacation or on a business trip? Make room in your suitcase for your walking shoes, because there's no better way to experience a new place than on foot. Whether you find yourself in a new city by chance or you've decided you want to explore locales that are great for walkers, make a plan to get the most of your visit by hoofing it.

Top 10 Walking Vacation Destinations

There are some places you need only see once. Las Vegas and Niagara Falls come to mind. There are other places you want to visit again and again, because you feel as if there's so much to see and do and you just can't get enough. These destinations are usually appealing because you can really get to know the place and experience it like a local—on foot. Below are 10 of the all-time most walk-worthy destinations in

America, from great cities like New York, Chicago, and Seattle to treasured national parklands like Acadia National Park in Maine or the Tahoe Rim Trail in Lake Tahoe, Nevada. Fly or drive to get there, then lace up your walking shoes and have the time of your life.

New York, New York

A walking vacation in the Big Apple is the only way to go. Every neighborhood is its own destination; around every corner a new experience awaits. From historic Harlem to Central Park, from the Great White Way to Ground Zero, from the fabled Bronx to trendy Brooklyn, from glitzy Fifth Avenue to gritty Greenwich Village, you could spend a week trekking New York City and still not see it all.

Are you a movie buff? Tour the locations of your favorite film scenes. Are you a foodie? Traipsing around Little Italy, Chinatown, and Tribeca will work up your appetite. Rock music lovers can make a walking pilgrimage to the neighborhoods that the Ramones, Bob Dylan, and Blondie called home or the storied venues where the Doors or the Who played late into the night. Just be sure to wear a pedometer; you'll be shocked at the miles you log even in a single day in New York. It may be the city that never sleeps, but it's also the city that walks—a lot.

San Francisco, California

EVEN IF YOU'RE PRESSED FOR TIME, TRY TO SQUEEZE IN A WALK WHEN YOU'RE TRAVELING.

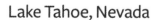

With multiple neighborhoods featuring world-class shops, restaurants, parks, museums, and other local attractions, San Francisco is recognized as a "walker's paradise." The city's particular distinction is the terrain—specifically, the more than 50 hills within city limits that can make going to the neighborhood coffee shop a heart-thumping workout. Visit Chinatown, Haight-Ashbury, Nob Hill, Telegraph Hill,

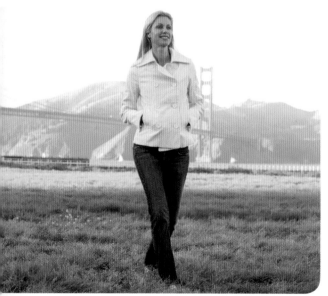

Pacific Heights, the Financial District, and North Beach—hey, and you may as well take a few steps around Alcatraz while you're there, right?

Take a Painted Ladies tour of the city's colorful Victorian landmark homes. Or take a leisurely all-day walk along the Embarcadero, from Fisherman's Wharf to the Ferry Plaza Farmer's Market to AT&T Park, to catch a Giants game. The fact is, you can easily drive around in San Francisco, but why would you want to?

Lake Tahoe, Nevada

The Tahoe Rim Trail features 96 miles of recreational trail across the ridges that surround the Lake Tahoe Basin. Gorge yourself on views of the lake, mountains, forests, and wildflower-filled meadows on the 65-mile East Trail, which wends through state park and national forest land and mountain passes straight out of an old Western. The 31-mile North Trail features miles of woodland punctuated with breathtaking views of the lake and surrounding mountains, crosses the Truckee River, passes a sweet waterfall near Ward Creek, and ends at Twin Peaks (not that Twin Peaks), California. If your hoofs get tired, maybe you can hitch a ride with one of the horseback riders or bicyclists with whom you'll be sharing this spectacular trail.

Boston, Massachusetts

We call it the Freedom Trail now, centuries after the founding of Boston in 1630. But our forefathers (and mothers) just called it home in the earliest days of the republic. Today the 2½-mile walk through time passes fabled landmarks, including Faneuil Hall, the King's Chapel, and the Old South Meeting House, as well as the Boston Common, the Massachusetts State House, and the U.S.S. *Constitution*. Depending on what time of year you visit, you can also see Revolutionary War reenactments, military parades, fireworks, concerts, and ceremonies honoring Revolutionary War heroes like Samuel Adams and John Hancock. Turn up on the 4th of July and you'll catch the reading of the Declaration of Independence from the balcony of the Old State House, an annual tradition that draws great crowds of patriots.

PLAN YOUR VACATIONS WITH FAMILY-FRIENDLY WALKS IN MIND.

Acadia National Park, Maine

A 10-hour drive from New York and six from Boston, it's a bit of a hike to get here. But the 120 miles of hiking trails for beginners and experienced hikers you find when you arrive make it more than worth the trip. The extraordinary terrain includes rugged coastline, pine woods, and granite peaks with views of the Atlantic Ocean and islands off the coast. There are also 45 miles of "carriage roads" for walking, bicycling, and horseback riding through some of the prettiest landscape east of the Mississippi. Visit in late September and catch the Acadia Night Sky Festival, which celebrates the brilliant celestial treasures of Acadia.

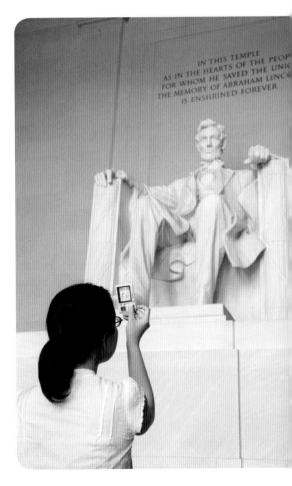

Washington, D.C.

From the steps of the U.S. Capitol to the Lincoln Memorial, at just shy of 2 miles, the National Mall is diminutive compared to other national parks. But given the proximity to an abundance of the country's most memorable monuments, museums, and gardens, as well as that famous residence at 1600 Pennsylvania Avenue, one could tour most of the nation's capital without ever leaving the Mall!

Create your own themed walking itineraries—do "The Presidents Walk," including visits to the White House, the Washington Monument, and the Lincoln, Jefferson, and FDR Memorials. Or spend an afternoon walking the World War II, Vietnam Veterans, and the Korean War Veterans memorials. Trek through tony Georgetown, take a jog along the Potomac on the Rock Creek Parkway, or walk straight up Connecticut Avenue, through the Dupont Circle and Adams Morgan neighborhoods, to get a good look at those Giant Pandas at the National Zoo. Prime time for walking Washington is early spring, of course, when the sun shines brightly, the air is cool and clear, and the cherry blossoms beckon.

Chicago, Illinois

The Windy City has got it all: the architecture and art, the food and shopping, the panoramic views of Lake Michigan, and the Bulls, Bears, Blackhawks, Cubs, and those rascally White Sox. And you can walk it from top to bottom and right to left. Wear yourself out at the world-famous Art Institute of Chicago, the Field Museum, and the Shedd Aquarium, then take in all 24 acres of Millenium Park, which offers a wondrous display of architecture, sculpture, and landscape design. A walk around the Loop takes you through the historic commercial center of the city, including the theater, shopping, and financial districts, which feature the Chicago Board of Trade Building and the Sears Tower, among many other sites. And what walker could resist the fabled Magnificent Mile, that landmark stretch of Michigan Avenue known as one of the great shopping destinations of the world? It may be one of the world's great cities, but Chicago is also as friendly and walkable as any small town in America.

Seattle, Washington

Seattle is one of those places that people fall in love with. It's beautiful, livable, unbe-lievably temperate, and it's got all that great coffee. Oh, and it's one of America's great walking cities, too. From wherever you stand, it is likely you can see Elliot Bay, Puget Sound, and the Olympic Mountains or Lake Washington and the Cascade Mountains. An outdoorsy person's dream, Seattle boasts miles of parks and trails in and around the city, including Discovery Park, a 500+-acre urban oasis that features a 2.8-mile loop through native forests and meadows home to 150 species of wildlife and seacliff views of Puget Sound.

Neighborhood walks around the Pike Place Market, Pioneer Square, Seattle Center and Queen Anne Hill give an unforgettable taste of a city with an independent nature and a rich history. Seattle is hilly, though, especially in the city center, which is proba-bly why natives generally forgo the Manolos in favor of a comfy pair of walking shoes.

JOIN THE CLUB

Walking with other people is good for you. When you walk with a buddy, you get not only the health benefits but also the social and motivational advantages. If you really want to up the ante, hook up with a walking club. Check with a walking organization such as the International Volkssport Association (IVV) to see if there's a walking club near you. Check also at the local health club or even your nearest mall.

If you can't find one, start one! Organize a walking group through Meetup.com to make it easy to communicate. Advertise for walkers at local schools, malls, or churches. Once you gather a nice crew, set up a schedule for different lengths and types of walks. Ask for volunteers to lead the various walks or to organize the group for walking events. And be sure to schedule social time outside of your organized walks. A nice picnic or breakfast together once a month will keep the group on a happy path.

Finally, whether you just walk with a regular partner or hoof with a whole group, keep these guidelines in mind:

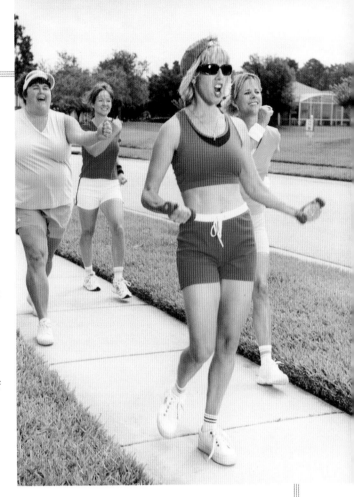

Be there, and be on time.

Don't flake out on your co-walkers by showing up late or not showing up at all. Do it more than once and you'll soon be walking solo.

Have a plan.

Agree on the distance in advance and how difficult your walk will be. Walkers that aren't walking at the same pace aren't walking together, right?

Establish friendly ground rules.

What if you want to listen to your MP3 but your partner wants to talk? Or your partner likes to bring her dog along? It helps to know your walking friend well enough to be able to say, "Can you let me know when you're thinking of bringing Fido?" or "Do you mind if I listen to some music for a while?" If you don't, though, be direct about your preferences. Setting a rule about cell phones—say, ringer off; answer only if it's your kids—is always a good idea.

Watch what you say.

Just because you're spending an hour a day with someone doesn't mean they need to know about your personal problems or other complaints. They also probably don't need to know how you feel about religion or politics, either. Sharing too much information will likely cause an uncomfortable dynamic somewhere down the road, so just don't.

Work a walk-a-thon.

A great way to get focused on fitness and do some good at the same time is to participate in a walkathon. You will likely have to plan and train for the event, which is a great motivator, and it's great to do with family and friends, especially for a cause you're passionate about. Walkathons are not just fun and games, however. The Avon Walk for Breast Cancer, for example, is a nearly 40-mile, two-day walk for which organizers recommend participants begin training up to 19 weeks in advance. You can easily find a worthy charity to put your steps behind or you can organize a walkathon yourself, as a fundraiser for your church or your kid's school, for example. Go to www.thewalkingsite.com/events to locate a walkathon near you or go to www.walkathon-guide.com for great info on planning an event.

Gettysburg, Pennsylvania

You don't have to be a Civil War buff to appreciate the experience of walking the site of the Battle of Gettysburg, where in July of 1863, Major General George Gordon Meade's Army of the Potomac defeated General Robert E. Lee's Army of Northern Virginia, ending General Lee's invasion of the North and providing the turning point of the Civil War. Nearly 50,000 soldiers from both sides died in the three-day battle. Some four months later President Abraham Lincoln delivered his historic Gettysburg Address at the dedication of the Soldiers' National Cemetery there.

Stop at the National Park Service Museum and visitors center and grab a map for the 6-hour, 10-mile Billy Yank Trail or the 2½-hour, 4-mile Johnny Reb Trail hikes through the battlefield, which are designed to give walkers the soldier's perspective over those three dark days. An added bonus? While dogs are normally prohibited from national park trails, they are generally welcome at historical parks and battle-fields. So by all means, bring Fido along!

Summertime can be quite crowded at Gettysburg, so go in the spring, when apple blossoms are in glorious abundance or in fall, when you can eat some of those apples!

Minneapolis, Minnesota

Known as one of America's most walkable cities, Minneapolis doesn't disappoint. For starters, its 8-mile "skyway" system—the largest in the world—of glass tunnels one story above the ground lets you get just about anywhere downtown in climate-controlled comfort every season of the year. Depending on how you plan it, you could see and do everything you want to on a cold day in January wearing just your shirtsleeves!

Sophisticated architecture, arts, and culture blend into the lushness of the land-scape, from the extensive green park system in the heart of the city itself to the historic riverfront district, which features the Mill City Museum and Farmer's Market and the Stone Arch Bridge, among many other sites overlooking the mighty Missis-sippi River. And if it's a rainy day, take a 40-minute ride on the Hiawatha Light Rail to the Mall of America and hook up with the MOA Mall Stars walking club, which you can catch 364 days a year doing one of the mile, 5K, or 10K mall walks mapped out by the Mayo Clinic.

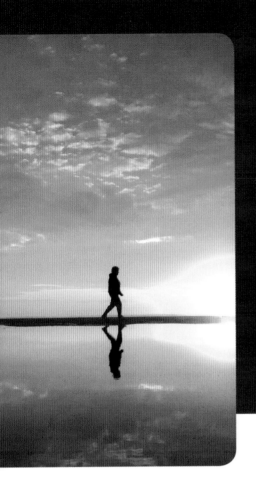

More Grounds for Walking

You're a real walker now—someone who walks on purpose, for fitness, for fun, and because it comes naturally to a happy, healthy body. You know why to walk, how to walk, and where to walk. You know all the tricks to get the best workout from your walk and how to avoid injuries and other trouble. The only thing missing, perhaps, from your walking lifestyle is a way of thinking about walking that isn't about the step-by-step of losing weight, but focuses instead on the other amazing things that can happen when you walk. Here are 10 "walks with benefits" to inspire you.

The God Walk

Spiritual contemplation doesn't have to take place in church. This weekend take a long walk in the big cathedral that's all around you—it's called Planet Earth.

First step—Think about what you're thankful for, or dedicate the time to thinking about a loved one or someone who's struggling. Solitary, mindful walking can be as meditative as prayer.

The Reverse Walk

We are creatures of habit. Break yours by occasionally walking your normal route in the other direction. It not only beats boredom but it'll wake you up to the world around you by helping you see things from fresh angles.

First step—Go left instead of right when you take your first step. Make a point to notice three things you never noticed from the opposite direction. And don't forget how to get home.

The Going Nowhere Fast Walk

EXERCISE
GUARANTEES EACH
OTHER'S UNDIVIDED
ATTENTION.

For those days when the weather is bleak or your schedule is even bleaker, make your way to the gym or the spare bedroom for a treadmill walk. Instead of being bored because you're, well, on a treadmill, turn these walks into another kind of adventure.

First step—Get a large-scale map of your state or some exotic country. After each workout, highlight the distance you've covered across your map. The next time someone asks how you got into such great shape, answer, "By walking the Appalachian Trail!"

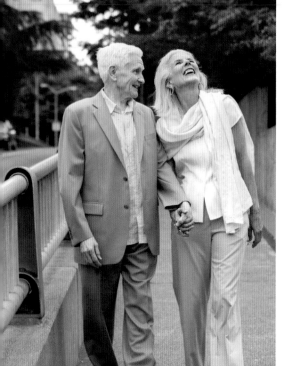

The Better Marriage Walk

Worried that you and your mate don't talk anymore? Walking together can help. Exercise makes us more open, emotional, and honest, plus it guarantees each other's undivided attention.

First step—Keep it low-key to start. Talk about things you notice along the way, interesting items in the news, etc. Then once your partner's warmed up, broach the more serious stuff. Hold hands. If you're lucky, this outing may morph into...

The Better Sex Walk

Believe it or not, the tongue is the most important sex organ. Communication promotes closeness. Plus, exercise naturally spikes libido by making us more aware of our bodies and helping us feel better about ourselves.

First step—Work up a sweat. That healthy glow is sexy. And don't be shy about occasionally talking suggestively. You'll both pick up the pace as you make the turn for home.

The Gripe Walk

When something is really getting on your nerves, hit the road instead of the wall. You'll not only get a great physical workout because the adrenaline will naturally make you walk faster, you'll also burn off some of the stress hormones coursing through your body.

First step—Don't rant or fume, just walk long and hard enough to let off the steam that wants to make your head pop off your neck.

Try to redirect your thoughts to something peaceful or pleasing to you. When all else fails, careful breathing (in one-two-three-four, out one-two-three-four) can bring you back to your senses.

The Rainy Day Walk

At the first sign of precipitation, many people go into hibernation. But there's something about walking in the rain that is simultaneously calming and exhilarating.

First step—Leave the umbrella at home. Instead, put on your waterproof shoes and a slicker with a hood. Every once in a while, tip your head back and catch a few raindrops on your tongue. It's a tonic.

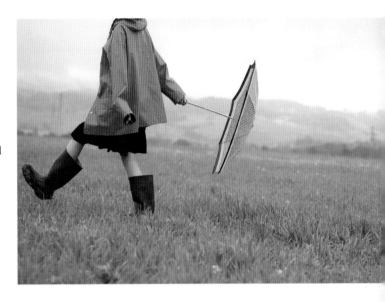

The Sleep Walk

Most Americans are chronically sleep deprived. In fact, many of us, because of stress and caffeine, have become incapable of getting the restful zzzzz's we need. Walking is one of the best ways to relax and set yourself up for a good night's sleep.

First step—Schedule your walk for between 4 and 7 P.M. Your body temperature is highest then, your muscles are warmest, and you'll have plenty to mull over from the day. The resulting calm will help you drift off at bedtime and sustain good sleep throughout the night.

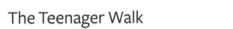

THERE'S NO NEED TO GO INTO HIBERNATION AT THE FIRST SIGN OF PRECIPITATION.

The Teenager Walk

This is one of the world's best ways to get that uncommunicative someone (your teenager) to open up.

First step—Tell your youthful ward that you're going to the supermarket and ask if he'd like to come along and pick out some food. (Teen metabolisms can't resist an offer like this.) When he heads for the car, tell him you're walking and invite him along. Bingo.

The Figure-It-Out Walk

There's something about putting one foot in front of the other that focuses the mind and brings clarity. A problem that might have overwhelmed you initially or one that appeared to have no solution will often solve itself during a walk.

First step—Don't dwell on the problem. Instead, think about it to start, then let it go. Your subconscious will keep working on it, and before long, like magic, a solution will appear.

TEST YOUR WALKING SMARTS

So now you think you know everything there is to know about walking. We'll see about that. Even seasoned walkers don't always have all the facts. Test your knowledge by taking this quiz, then look at the opposite page to find some surprising answers. We guarantee you'll learn a thing or two.

1. **HOW MANY CALORIES DOES 1 MILE OF WALKING BURN?**
   - ☐ **a** 200
   - ☐ **b** 80
   - ☐ **c** 100

2. **TO WALK FASTER, INCREASE YOUR STRIDE LENGTH.**
   - ☐ **a** True
   - ☐ **b** False

3. **HOW LONG DO WALKING SHOES LAST?**
   - ☐ **a** 6 months to 1 year
   - ☐ **b** 1 to 2 years
   - **c** 3 years

4. **WHICH INCREASES YOUR CALORIE BURN THE MOST?**
   - ☐ **a** Walking uphill
   - ☐ **b** Wearing a backpack
   - ☐ **c** Carrying hand weights

5. **"GAIT SPEED" IS A KEY INDICATOR OF:**
   - ☐ **a** Low mortality rate
   - ☐ **b** Leg strength
   - ☐ **c** Lung capacity

6. **WHAT IS AN "AVERAGE" WALKING PACE?**
   - ☐ **a** 3 m.p.h.
   - ☐ **b** 1 m.p.h.
   - ☐ **c** 2 m.p.h.

7. **HOW MANY MILES DO YOU NEED TO WALK EACH WEEK TO CUT YOUR HEART ATTACK RISK IN HALF?**
   - ☐ **a** 12 to 14
   - ☐ **b** 5 to 6
   - ☐ **c** 8 to 10

8. **AFTER A BRISK 2-HOUR WALK YOUR BODY CONTINUES TO BURN CALORIES FOR HOW MANY HOURS?**
   - ☐ **a** 12
   - ☐ **b** 1
   - ☐ **c** 24

9. **EVERY MINUTE OF WALKING EXTENDS YOUR LIFE BY HOW MUCH?**
   - ☐ **a** 30 seconds
   - ☐ **b** 5 minutes
   - ☐ **c** 1.5 to 2 minutes

10. **WHICH BRAIN BENEFIT DOES WALKING NOT PROVIDE?**
    - ☐ **a** Better memory
    - ☐ **b** A higher IQ
    - ☐ **c** Improved problem-solving

11. **THE AVERAGE PERSON TAKES HOW MANY STEPS PER DAY?**
    - ☐ **a** 5,000 to 6,000
    - ☐ **b** 2,000 to 3,000
    - ☐ **c** 8,000 to 10,000

Answers

1. C 100 CALORIES

A person weighing 150 pounds burns about 100 calories every mile. Not a whole lot, but it isn't just calorie burn that's important. Walking builds metabolism-revving muscle tissue in your lower body, melts away dangerous belly fat (even if you don't lose much weight), and improves your heart health and fitness and energy levels, so you're more likely to keep moving—and combusting calories.

2. B FALSE

This is a common misconception among walkers of all experience levels, but especially beginners. Lengthening your stride may make you feel like you're covering more ground, but it actually slows you down, since your front foot lands outstretched like a brake, hampering your progress. It's also inefficient, so you fatigue faster. Instead, speed up by taking short, quick strides, concentrating on pushing off your toes with ever step. Hint: Pumping your arms quickly will automatically make your feet move faster.

3. A 6 MONTHS TO 1 YEAR

This answer is somewhat dependent upon how often you walk. Most shoes are built to last about 500 miles. After that, the cushioning breaks down, and your body starts absorbing the impact instead. If you're walking 30 or 40 minutes per day most days of the week, replace your shoes before a year is up. (To remember when you bought them, write the date on the inside of the tongue.)

4. B WEARING A BACKPACK

Wearing either a knapsack with a few books or other hefty items—like groceries inside or a weighted walking vest can nearly double your calorie burn, scorching about 475 calories per hour. Skip the hand weights. They may increase calorie burn, but they can strain shoulders, elbows, and wrists. Prefer to walk unencumbered? Hit the hills. Hoofing against gravity burns nearly as many calories as walking with extra weight.

5. A LOW MORTALITY RATE

How fast you walk is a strong indicator of your general health. In a recent study of walkers age 65-plus, researchers found that those who walked the fastest had lower mortality rates. The key speed for sidestepping ill health was at least 2.25 m.p.h. for people in this age group. Need a speed boost? Try some resistance training (especially squats) to improve leg strength. Also, add intervals to your fitness walks. Every 2 to 3 minutes, increase your pace above your comfort zone for 30 to 60 seconds. Eventually, your regular walking speed will rise, too.

6. C 2 M.P.H.

Most people naturally walk between 1.5 and 2.5 mph. That's fine for window-shopping, but if you want to lose weight and optimize fitness, aim higher. A good walking speed for fitness is 3 to 4 m.p.h.—the pace you walk when you're late for a meeting or cruising through the airport to make a flight.

7. A 12 TO 14 MILES

The Honolulu Heart Study found that men who walked about 2 miles per day had half the heart attack risk as their counterparts who walked a quarter mile or less. But even logging less mileage still has significant cardio benefits. The Nurse's Health Study of more than 72,000 women found that those who walked 1.3 miles per day (the equivalent of 9 miles per week at a 3-m.p.h. pace) reduced their heart attack risk by 35 percent.

8. A 12 HOURS

Kinesiologists—people who study body movement—determined that metabolism stays revved for a full 12 hours after a brisk 2-hour walk. That's another great reason to schedule long walks on the weekends.

9. C 1.5 TO 2 MINUTES

That's right, when it comes to lifespan, walking delivers a two-for-one special! If you ever doubted it in the past, here's proof that every minute of walking does indeed count.

10. B A HIGHER IQ

Okay, walking won't actually increase your intelligence. But it sure will make you feel smarter. In a study of more than 18,000 women age 70 and older, researchers found that those who walked at least 1.5 hours per week scored higher on tests of memory, general problem solving, and attention compared to those who walked less than 40 minutes per week. Walking also reduces your risk of developing dementia.

11. A 5,000 TO 6,000

That's about 3 miles (1 mile is about 2,000 steps). While that's enough to produce some measurable benefits—like cutting heart-attack risk—for optimum health and fitness, experts recommend taking 10,000 steps per day.

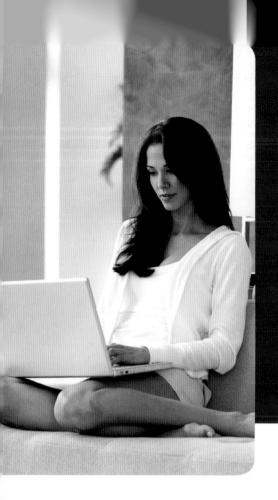

Great Gear to Step Out In

Below are some great sources for the clothes and other gear that can make walking more comfortable, safe, and fun.

Gadgets

Pedometers

The Yamax and Accusplit Digi-Walker Pedometers are inexpensive, accurate, and available at most sporting good stores. The Omron Digital Pocket Pedometer is an accurate, multi-functional pedometer that works just as well tucked in your pocket or handbag as it does clipped to your hip. All are available at www.pedometersusa.com. The Gaiam Pedometer Fit Kits (www.gaiam.com) are inexpensive combination pedometer-audio workout program sets for beginner, intermediate, and advanced level walkers.

Heart monitors

The Polar Activity Computer is a watch-style heart monitor that tracks calories burned, steps taken, distance traveled, and general activity level. It also lets you upload this information and track your progress on the Polar website. Go to (www.polarusea.com) to check it out. See also the highly accurate Sportline Solo watch-style combination heart monitor/pedometers (www.sportline.com), which also feature a timer for interval training and a backlit display that makes it easy to read on dawn or dusk walks.

Wrist Gear

If you want an easy way to carry just your essentials—house key, ID, cash, credit card, and lip balm—the Power Walkers Wrist Pocket is ideal. Made of polyester and spandex, it's stretchy and comfortable around your wrist and has a locking zip (www.walkwear.org).

For peace of mind, Road ID makes stylish ID wear engraved with your emergency contact information in case you are injured while walking and can't call for help on your own. Road ID produces wrist IDs, shoe IDs, and ankle IDs, which come in several colors and with two 3M reflective stripes to enhance your visibility when training in the dark (www.roadid.com).

GPS

For walking in the wild or otherwise unfamiliar places, the Original Bushnell Back-Track GPS Personal Location Finder is easy to use, conveniently sized, and also features a Boy Scout-worthy digital compass. (www.bushnellgps.com).

A GOOD BACKPACK SHOULD BE LIGHT-WEIGHT, STURDY, AND ABLE TO HOLD EVERY-THING YOU NEED.

MP3 accessories

The Sportline Walking Advantage MP3 holder is a flexible, padded armband carrier that fits and protects any size MP3 device, and also features reflective material that improves your visibility while walking day or night. (www.sportline.com). And if your earphones won't stay put when you walk, check out Skullcandy's Asym Earbuds, which feature little cables that hook over your ears to secure them in place. And because they sit flush to the outside of your ear, you can easily wear them under a cap. Awesome sound quality, too (www.skull-candy.com).

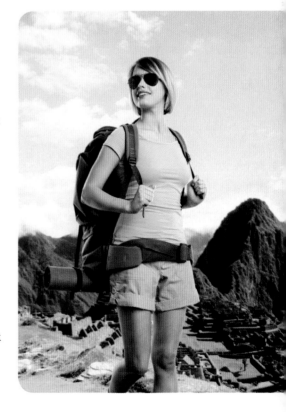

Equipment

Backpacks and waist packs

Camelbak produces top-knotch backpacks and waist packs in a variety of shapes and sizes for walkers, bikers, and hikers (www.camelbak.com). The compact Ultimate Direction Uno Hydration Pack (www.ultimatedirection.com) features zippered storage pockets for keys, cash, and ID—and comes with a BPA-free water bottle, too!

Walking poles

Leki and Black Diamond make a variety of top-quality walking poles, from performance poles for high-altitude trekking, lightweight and shock-absorbing fitness walking poles, and trail poles (www.leki.com and www.blackdiamondequipment.com). Look for adjustable length, anti-shock features, and a grip that's comfortable to you.

Water bottles

Camelbak's spillproof, BPA-free Better Bottles (www.camelbak.com) are, well, better! You can clip it to your beltloop or backpack or carry it on the crook of your finger.

Sunglasses

Zeal Optics makes top-drawer polarized, impact-resistant sports sunglasses (www.zealoptics.com). Even cooler, they also produce the Transcend GPS Goggle, which features built-in GPS for the off-the-grid adventurer. Smith Optics has a dazzling array of polarized, high-performance sports sunglasses (www.smithoptics.com), as does Suncloud Optics (www.suncloudoptics.com).

BEFORE YOU GO OUT AND BUY A NEW PAIR OF SNEAKERS , SEE PAGE 29 TO IDENTIFY WHAT KIND OF FEET YOU HAVE.

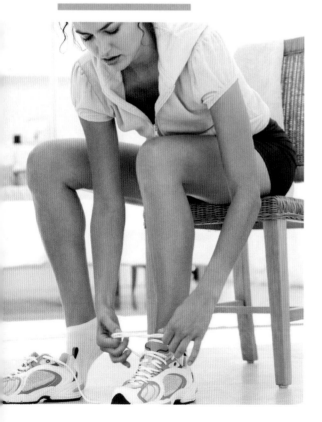

Clothes

There are several companies who produce high-quality clothes that are appropriate for multi-season walking. Check out Brooks (www.brooks.com) and Athleta (www.athleta.com) for a variety of fast-drying, easy-movement tees, tops, shorts and pants. REI (www.rei.com) L.L. Bean (www.llbean.com), and Northface (www.northface.com) will not disappoint with a variety of fleece vests and jackets, windbreakers, and light- and heavier-weight outerwear, among other great outdoor wear and gear. Illuminite makes an all-star adjustable cold-weather Therma Fleece cap (www.illuminite.com) that's got a bill and a flap in the back you can pull down to keep your neck warm. The fabric is also embedded with reflected particles, which makes this a great topper when walking at dawn or dusk.

Socks

Nike's DriFit socks (www.nike.com) are great for everyday walking, while Smartwool crew socks (www.smartwool.com) and Lorpen's mixed weight Tri-Layer socks (www.lorpen.com/lorpen-na) are great for hiking or cold weather.

Sneakers

You can choose among your favorite brands, from Asics (www.asicsamerica.com) and Nike (www.nike.com), to Saucony (www.saucony.com) and New Balance (www.new-balance.com), all of which produce sneakers designed specifically for walkers, and most of which also offer options for over- and under-pronators.

Hiking shoes

Keen Footwear makes outstanding waterproof hiking shoes, boots, and sandals (www.keenfootwear.com). Teva produces waterproof light hiking shoes made of breathable eVent material (www.teva.com). And if you want to give an ordinary walking shoe a little hiking boot cred, attach a pair of Yaktrax Pro to your soles (www.yaktrax.com). The instant traction you'll get on ice or snow is amazing.

Apps

The iTreadmill app for the iPod or iPhone is like a trainer in your pocket, using the motion detector in the device to help you measure pace and distance wherever and whenever you walk (www.iTreadmill.com).

WalkJogRun is an app that can help you map out a walking route just about any-where, whether it's a new city or your own hometown. You can browse routes by location and see estimates of the number of calories you'll burn on each route (www.walkjogrun.net).

The MapMyWalk app lets you search for an existing route or create and map your own. You can also set goals and record your progress through the website (www.mapmywalk.com).

RunKeeper uses GPS technology to track your distance, time, pace, calories burned, and the route you took. Your data then syncs to the RunKeeper website and helps you keep track of your progress (www.runkeeper.com).

Index

muscle(s). *See also specific kinds*
   building, 19
   cramps in, 105
   rubbing, 105
   soreness in, 104–5
   tension, 16
   toning exercises for, 70–71
   types of, 18
music
   country, 65
   hip-hop, 76
   moving to, 67
   R&B, Rock, 66
   soul, 46

N

naringenin, 126–27
neck, stretches for, 101
neighborhood beautification, walking and, 51
neurotransmitters, 73
New York, New York, 200
night-on-the-town, steps equated with, 23
non-exercise activity thermogenesis (NEAT), 81
Nordic walking technique, 62
nuts, 117

O

oatmeal, 137
oats, 124
oblique muscles, toning exercises for, 71
omega-3 fatty acids, 125, 126
outdoor walking, 37–38
overhead stretch warm-up, 45

P

pacing, hikes and, 184
pain, 104–7
Park Presses (toning exercise), 70
Partial Lunge (exercise), 89
Partial Squat (exercise), 89

pears, 127
pedometers, 22–23, 62, 82, 210
Pelvic Twist Stretch, 91
peppers, sweet, 127
phosphorus, 73
pillows, 74
plank exercises, 192–93
Plank Glute Press (exercise), 193
Plank Twist (exercise), 192
plans
   dinner, 57
   8-week, 52–63
   interval workouts, 66–69
   for starting to walk, 46–49
plantar fasciitis, 106
playlists
   country music, 65
   hip-hop music, 76
   R&B music, 46
   Rock music, 66
   soul music, 46
Pole Side Pulls (toning exercise), 70
pollen count, 36
pork tenderloin preparation, 169
portion control, 112
posture, 95
potassium, 105
power foods, 122–28
power surge walking, 76
Prayer Pose (stretch), 103
prioritizing walking, 56
probiotics, 197
problem-solving, walking and, 51, 207
programs, walking, 46–49
protein, 57, 123, 124, 125, 126
purposeful walking, 50–51
pyramid walking, 76

Q

quad stretch warm-ups, 45
quick-step weight loss, 65–66
quinoa, 125, 149
quiz, 208–9

R

R&B music playlist, 46
racewalking, 65–66
Rag Doll to Open Arms (stretch), 101
rain, walking in, 33–34, 207
recipes, 132–79. *See also* Recipe Index, 219
rehearsals, walking and, 51
relaxing before eating, 115
resistance training, 19
resources, 210–13
reversing direction of walk, 206
Rhodiola rosea, 74
roseroot, 74

S

safety, 28, 184
salads, 113
saline nasal spray, 197
salmon, omega-3 fats and, 126
salt in foods, 117
San Francisco, California, 200
Scorpion (stretch), 103
seasons, 182–98
   socks and, 32
Seated Torso Twist stretch, 93
Seattle, Washington, 202
sedentary living, 15, 22
selenium, 126
Self-Hug (stretch), 96
serotonin, 16, 113, 115
serving suggestion, 112
sex, 83, 206
sherry vinegar, 152
shin splints, 107
shoes, 27, 28–30, 44
   for hiking, 184, 185, 212–13
   shin splits and, 107
   for winter, 196
shopping
   for groceries, 57, 114
   steps equated with, 23
shopping malls for walking, 39

Recipe Index

Credits

CONTRIBUTING WRITERS

Christie Aschwanden, Karen Asp, Alisa Bowman, Sari Harrar, John Hastings, David Joachim, Joe Kita, Dana Sullivan, Selene Yeager

Also Available from Reader's Digest

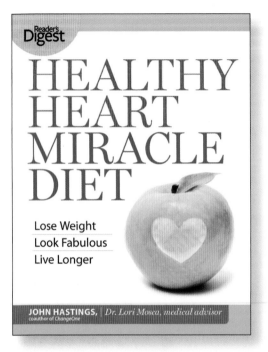

Healthy Heart Miracle Diet

This comprehensive guide will help you slim down, look terrific, and even add years to your life by delivering the final word on fat, complex and simple carbs, exercise, supplements, and more. Over 500 hints and tips clear up confusing nutritional claims, explode myths, and explain how eating right can be as easy as pie.

John Hastings
Lori Mosca, MD, Medical Advisor
978-1-60652-412-1
$17.99 U.S.A. paperback

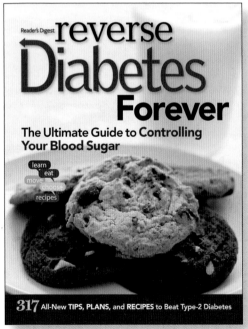

Reverse Diabetes Forever

Take control and reverse diabetes once and for all with simple exercises, diet-friendly meals, stress-reduction tips, recuperative sleep techniques, and lifestyle improvements. More than 50 exciting, easy recipes will ensure that you'll never be bored at mealtime again. With this handy companion your blood sugar numbers will start to plummet in no time!

From the Editors at Reader's Digest
978-1-60652-425-1
$17.99 U.S.A. paperback